THE GREAT BRITISH CORONAVIRUS HOAX

A Sceptic's Guide

By Nick Kollerstrom

The idea of quarantining millions of perfectly healthy people and stopping them from doing normal, healthy things is something that has apparently never occurred to any national leaders in the past. Rob Slane

ISBN: 978-1-9161821-4-1

A New Alchemy Press publication, 2020

Acknowledgements:

Thanks to Arthur Firstenberg for permission to use his text & to *UK Column* for permission to use their bar-chart; to *Spiked* online for use of their Wittkowski interview and to Janine Roberts for excepts from her book *Fear of the Invisible*. I'm grateful to members of the London Keeptalking group for stimulating discussions and much of the information used here, to Kevin Boyle for the Coronavirus Act section (Chapter Two), to Stephen Windsor-Clive for editorial advice, and to Simon Day and Joanna van der Leer for cover design.

Chronicle of Events

2018   January   China's first maximum security virology lab. opens in Wuhan.

November   The Pirbright Institute, Woking, issues patent for Coronavirus

2019   May   Swine fever hits China pig farms, 400m die

Aug 13   *Operation Crimson Contagion* held in Washington DC

Sept 12   Global Vaccination Summit held in Brussels

Sept 19   'ID2020' Alliance summit held in New York to promote 'digital identity'

Oct 1   'most recent common ancestor' claimed for the CV-19   RNA sequence in Wuhan

Oct 18-27   Military World Games held in Wuhan, China

Oct 18   *Event 201* held at John Hopkins University

Oct 31 1st 'large-scale 5G network engineering program' turned on in Wuhan

Nov   CEPI pledges $700m for development of DNA/RNA vaccines, especially against 'Disease X, a novel or unanticipated pathogen'

Dec 2   Two-day Global Vaccine Safety Summit in Geneva by the WHO

Dec 31   China reports first CV-19 infection, and alerts WHO to the virus.

2020 Jan 12   Chinese publish complete genome of the virus

Jan 20 Netflix releases *Pandemic: how to Prevent an Outbreak*

Jan 23   Lockdown & quarantine of entire city of Wuhan

Jan 23   CEPI announces initiation of programs to develop CV-19 vaccine

Mar 5   Ist British death CV+

Mar 17   Prof Ferguson at Imperial College predicts half a million UK CV-19 deaths.

Mar 17   French lockdown

Mar 23   British Lockdown

CEPI – The Coalition for Epidemic Preparedness Innovations

Contents

Author's works

Terror on the Tube, Behind the Veil of 7/7 an Investigation 2009
The Life and Death of Paul McCartney 1942-66 a very English
Mystery   2015
How Britain Initiated both World Wars   2017
False Flags over Europe   A Modern History of State-fabricated
Terror   2018
Who did 9/11? A View from Across the Pond   2018
The Great British Skripal Hoax   2019
The Novichok Chronicles A Tale of Two Hoaxes   2020
     For other books by NK see his Amazon author's page

Note for 2nd Edition: I have left chapters 1-7 more or less
unchanged, merely adding on a couple of extra chapters.

1

The Hoax

Spring Equinox 2020: Unprecedented lockdown orders are given out right across the UK. No you can't take your dog for a walk. Schools close, shops close and everyone learns about 'social distancing.' There is some deadly new bug around, isn't there?

Several days prior to March 23rd, when the decision was made, the government was given some high-level medical advice so let's take a look at it.[1] The same day March 23rd its website stated:

> As of 19 March 2020, COVID-19 is no longer considered to be a high consequence infectious diseases (HCID) in the UK.

It explained:

> The 4 nations public health HCID group made an interim recommendation in January 2020 to classify COVID-19 as an HCID. This was based on consideration of the UK HCID criteria about the virus and the disease with information available during the early stages of the outbreak. Now that more is known about COVID-19, the public health bodies in the UK have reviewed the most up to date information about COVID-19 against the UK HCID criteria. They have determined that several features have now changed; in particular, more information is available about mortality rates (low overall).

This was a big step and a rather sensible one. Initially a group of four nations had been persuaded to agree, that a new 'high consequence infectious disease' existed. Everyone was terrified by what had been happening in Wuhan, China, and the possibility of it

---

1 Jointly produced by Public Health England (PHE) and the Advisory Committee on Dangerous Pathogens (ACDP).

spreading overseas. Had it not arrived already? What was 'it'? But then 'now that more was known about COVID-19' by reviewing the most up-to-date information, a revision of the early judgment was deemed appropriate, by those concerned to protect public health. And one prime factor is mentioned, as affecting that revision, which was that 'more information is available about mortality rates (low overall).'

Let's have a look at the evidence that the top government experts were perusing, on that fateful spring equinox. This must be a rational process, based on empirical evidence. Whereas, on the contrary, the massive decision HMG made on that very day flew absolutely in the face of this new and carefully-phased advice. That is what we will explore here. You are invited to judge for yourself whether or not the word 'hoax' is appropriate. Is there any possible rational explanation, as to why HMG went immediately into the most draconian lockdown? It could perhaps have said HMG needs a few days to evaluate and take advice following this major downgrading of the danger or otherwise, of this frightening new threat.

There does not exist in the UK anything resembling an EPA, Environmental Protection Agency, any national body concerned with the heath of the population against ambient threats such as pollution or radiation. I always find this hard to believe. For example are you concerned that 5G might be bad for your health? Or maybe, bad for All Life on Earth? If so do not expect any national body to be capable of reviewing evidence in this respect: no, one just has to find a few elderly retired persons who have worked in the electronics industry who are (if we're lucky) prepared to speak out, and who are old enough not to be intimidated by threats of job loss etc.

Supposing you wished to ask for example, 'Does a "COVID-19" virus exist?' What is meant by saying that? For example, is anyone claiming to have seen it down an electron microscope or to have

<u>Figure</u>: Dettol disinfectant bottle, showing how it claims to zap 'human coronavirus'

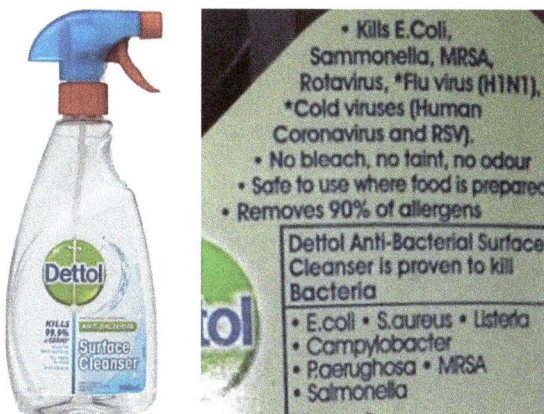

sequenced its genetic structure? In raising such queries, you'll soon find yourself labelled as a conspiracy theorist. Oh you're one of those are you? On some 'conspiracy' sites one can read about how coronaviruses are a normal component of the flu viruses that sweep around the world every year, and whether or not this one might be more deadly. All our lives we had been told there could not be a vaccine against the flu, because vaccines apply to bacteria which are alive and not to viruses which are not; and because viruses mutate all the

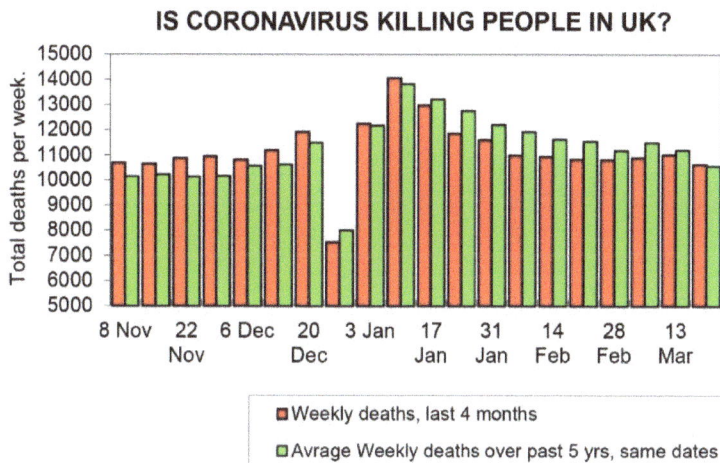

IS CORONAVIRUS KILLING PEOPLE IN UK?

Weekly deaths, last 4 months

Avrage Weekly deaths over past 5 yrs, same dates

time, they do not have a fixed form that is stable for long enough. Our understanding of science tends to break down at this point, and media hype takes over.

In this chapter we won't go into theoretical issues such as whether a vaccine could exist against CV-19. Instead, we take a look at the overall data which the ONS Office of National Statistics have been providing, for weekly mortality data England and Wales. If some sort of dreadful pandemic is taking place such that you can't go to your gym or church or park, then it ought to show up in the figures, should it not?

The ONS publishes its data on www.ons.gov.uk and the page is called 'ALL DEATHS IN ENGLAND AND WALES (All cause mortality) by week, comparing 2020 with the previous 5 years'[2] Here it is as a bar-chart. The ONS gives us the total deaths per week, and also helpfully gives an average of the previous five years, of the same total weekly deaths. The CV scare hit the UK around the beginning of January. We can see over the weeks leading up to the Spring Equinox, how total deaths for 2020 were consistently *lower.* Overall since mid-January they have been 5% less. If you want to count them up, the from the week ending 17 January to the week ending 13th of March – that is nine weeks – there had been 5,175 LESS deaths in England and Wales, that the average of previous years. That is the first important piece of information which the government medical advisors would have scrutinised.

The festive season is having a big effect here as we can see: a regular deficit exists over the Xmas week, as if people don't want to die then, whereas over the gloomy start to the new year, mortality normally peaks in the first week of January. This doesn't concern us

---

2 Its URL is:
www.ons.gov.uk/peoplepopulationandcommunity/birthsdeathsandmarriages/deaths/dat asets/weeklyprovisionalfiguresondeathsregisteredinenglandandwales Click on a year to get an Excel spreadsheet with the data.

**Total weekly mortality England & Wales
as a % of previous 5 years, mean**

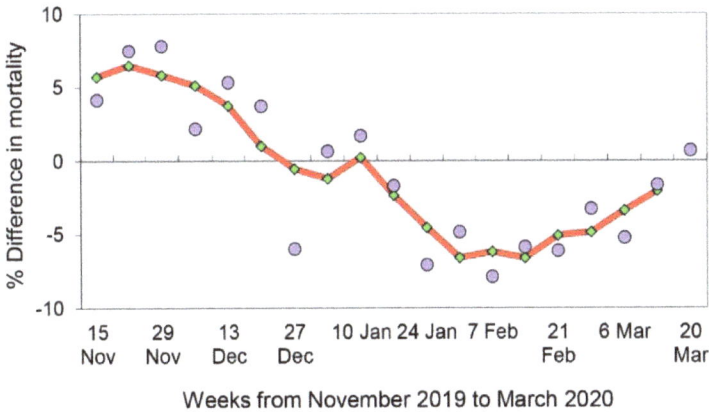

Weeks from November 2019 to March 2020

here but we just take note.

It is helpful to have the percentage differences for each week, of these two groups compiled by the ONS. I've put a trend-line (three-point moving average) through the data. We see the huge and rather puzzling swing, from an excess of deaths before Xmas to a deficit afterwards.

Also, very helpfully, that same ONS page gives weekly mortality for lung-related illnesses, what it calls 'deaths where the underlying

**Weekly lung-related deaths, total
England and Wales**

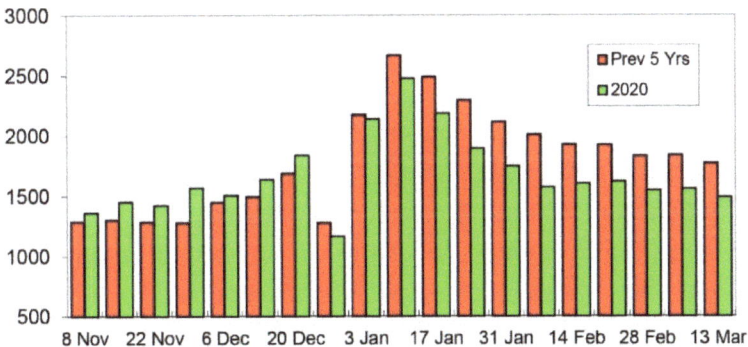

November 2019 - March 2020

cause was respiratory disease.' We've all heard harrowing stories about how hospitals are chock-a-block with patients on ventilators caused by this new pandemic, so that there are not enough hospital beds and large extra rooms and spaces have to be requisitioned. That should show up in the figures, shouldn't it?

But instead this new graph shows a staggering *decrease* in lung-related deaths in England and wales for all the months of this year. Given this data, how can anyone keep a straight face while claiming that some dreadful new lung-related pandemic is raging, enough to lock up the entire population in their rooms? It's deviation from the mean is three times *larger* than the previous total-death effect, with between 15% or 17% *less* dying! And this was for every week without exception! Here is the same data as we saw before but just plotting the percent difference each week:

Weekly lung-related deaths as % of mean from past 5 years

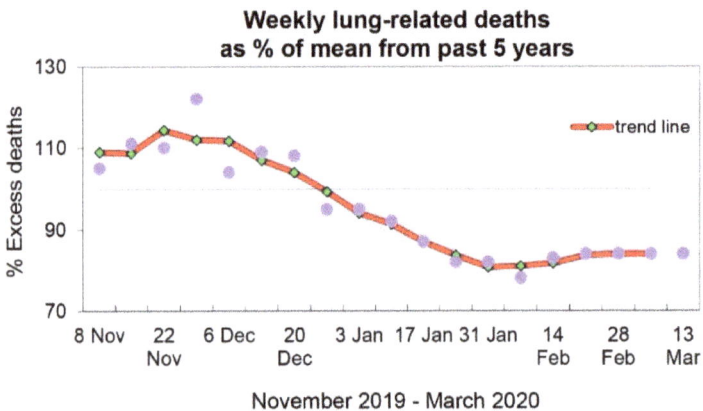

November 2019 - March 2020

After that 13th of March date, the ONS created a new category, of deaths where testing-positive-for-coronavirus goes onto the death certificate. Some of those will be cases where lung disease would otherwise have been regarded as the cause of death.

The ONS data we've now reviewed would have been the information about 'mortality rates (low overall)' that was presented to HMG by its medical experts on 19th of March. But in addition, they would have considered the global picture, which would have appeared somewhat as follows:

This showed that, over a three-month period, deaths 'by Coronavirus' (ie where a positive-result Cv-19 test was registered before death) were then on a global scale for instance fifty-four times *less* than deaths due to smoking; twelve times *less* than death by suicide, etc., and far less than for seasonal flu deaths. Does that sound like a major global 'pandemic'?

Roughly twenty thousand die each year on the UK from flu, or slightly less say seventeen thousand, over the past five years. Nobody fusses about that, we just accept it. Its mainly old people, and folk have to die of something. At the time of the government lockdown decision, CV-linked deaths were about half of one percent of that figure.

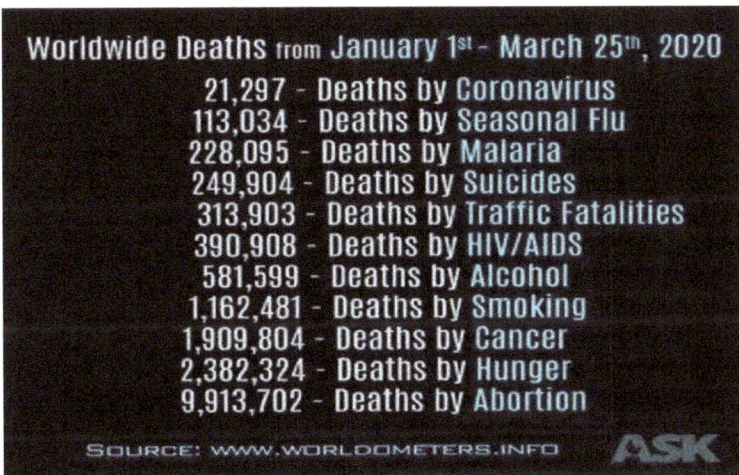

Worldwide Deaths from January 1st - March 25th, 2020

21,297 - Deaths by Coronavirus
113,034 - Deaths by Seasonal Flu
228,095 - Deaths by Malaria
249,904 - Deaths by Suicides
313,903 - Deaths by Traffic Fatalities
390,908 - Deaths by HIV/AIDS
581,599 - Deaths by Alcohol
1,162,481 - Deaths by Smoking
1,909,804 - Deaths by Cancer
2,382,324 - Deaths by Hunger
9,913,702 - Deaths by Abortion

SOURCE: WWW.WORLDOMETERS.INFO   ASK

These four items of information would have all been available and scrutinised, by the government's medical experts. Does not the decision made seem to have been *despite* the evidence, as if a pre-set agenda were being implemented? People are made to live in fear – a central principal of government in this 21st century - and the point here is that fear can override rational judgment. The phrase 'fear porn' has been developed by Olé Dammegard in this context, of how the Globalists (Bill Gates et. al.) keep catering for the public's expectation of a 'worse tomorrow' by generating images of fear and fabricated terror.

I'm suggesting that on that date the evidence in front of the government experts was so overwhelmingly against the decision they made, that one is justified in using the term 'hoax.' In subsequent chapters I will try to argue that a *globalist agenda* is playing out here. This is terribly important for anyone concerned with sovereignty. Is this country capable of making its own decisions in its own best interests? Or are its centres of expertise and decision-making to be just swept away by the tsunami of fear and alarm – we must act quickly! Quickly, give up all your democratic rights and decisions…don't worry you will get them back later on .. someday … if you're lucky.

Here are two opposite views on what might or might not be going on. Firstly, here is the aged Henry Kissinger, skilfully conjuring up the delusional fear-image:

> The reality is the world will never be the same after the coronavirus…. The coronavirus has struck with unprecedented scale and ferocity. Its spread is exponential. U.S. cases are doubling every fifth day. At this writing, there is no cure…. We live in an epochal period…. Failure could set the world on fire. – Henry Kissinger (The *Wall Street Journal* April 3rd)

How frightening! But, is that really happening? Or, an opposite view by a medical expert: 'If you want to create a totally false panic, about a totally false pandemic, pick a coronavirus' –

> Before long you have your pandemic, totally fabricated. All you've done is use a single test-kit trick to convert the worst flu and pneumonia cases into something new that

8

that doesn't actually exist. Now just run the same scam in other countries. Make sure to keep the fear running high so people will feel panicky and less able to think critically (Why COVID-19 is a scam designed to damage global economies.[3]

Could it be that *the test itself is generating the pandemic,* or rather the semblance of one? That would be a diabolically clever wheeze … but what would be the point? Governments should be slow to move on the great issues where the health of the population is involved; panic is the worst thing because it will very likely lead to a wrong course of action. If the population is drenched in fear – from watching too many horror movies, and expecting them to become true or in some degree actualised – calm rational discussion is hardly feasible. Your view becomes enormously important if the government experts have got it wrong.

On March 17th, Professor Neil Ferguson at Imperial college, London, scared everyone with a computer model showing the 'exponential' growth etc and that panicked the government 'experts' into the lockdown decision. It predicted that half a million UK citizens were going to die and globally, forty million people would die, unless something was done! Quickly, we'd better move! His model gave predictions about how healthcare systems were likely to be overwhelmed etc. and has been described as the 'ground zero for this world lockdown.' *As soon as* the lockdown measures were implemented then the day after he drastically revised his figures: no wait, it would only be twenty thousand… His unit receives funding from the Bill and Melinda Gates Foundation.

We will meet professor Ferguson later on, and see how the major US 'Event 201' - which gave a frame to the whole pandemic concept weeks before the 'real thing' hit the headlines – was put into action via his team at Imperial College. That receives tens of millions of

---

3 Jerry Day: it was up on .www.153news.net for7 April but that entire, very large site has been deleted.

dollars yearly from the Gates Foundation. It is also relevant that the Bill and Melinda Gates Foundation are major stakeholders of the Pirbright Institute in Woking, which came out with a patent for the (or, 'a') coronavirus in 2018.

The thirty-one authors of that Imperial College paper were advocating an 18-month lockdown ... just the same period as Bill Gates was advocating, *until* the vaccine was ready.

On that same date March 17th, the following mild and rather sensible comment appeared:

US010130701B2

10

If we had not known about a new virus out there, and had not checked individuals with PCR tests, the number of total deaths due to "influenza-like illness" would not seem unusual this year. At most, we might have casually noted that flu this season seems to be a bit worse than average.[4]

These are two very opposite views. Are we all conditioned to prefer fear and panic? The quiet, sensible and (I'd say) correct view is ignored by the media. Through a glorious springtime, the drug of fear blocks out normal critical-intellectual activity (frontal lobes of the cerebral cortex) replacing it by more primitive fight-and-flight behavior. And with that we saw the toilet rolls flying off the shelves!

After the Lockdown

Once the draconian and unprecedented lockdown was in place and everyone was 'social distancing,' would that affect total mortality? Suppose a massive surge in deaths occurred immediately *after* doing that, what would it show? Because that is certainly what did happen. Here is a helpful graph which the *Daily Mirror* published on 14th April.

It used exactly the same ONS figures we've used here, and sensibly subtracted the five-year weekly means from this year's data, showing how there was a deficit of deaths UNTIL the lockdown occurred. Then suddenly a massive surge took place, manly from COVID cases but also about 40% of the increase was from other deaths. If we take the two weeks before the lockdown compared to the two weeks after, the latter had *nearly forty times more* CV-related deaths. As you can see from the graph, that is a fantastic increase. We can all speculate why this should be, and how people

---

4 "A fiasco in the making? As the coronavirus pandemic takes hold, we are making decisions without reliable data", *Stat News*, 17th March Dr John Ioannidis Professor of Medicine, of Health Research and Policy and of Biomedical Data Science, at Stanford University School of Medicine, quoted in the Off-Guardian '12 Experts question the CV Panic'

**Death registrations in 2020 minus 5–year average
(ONS England+Wales, not necessarily week of death)**

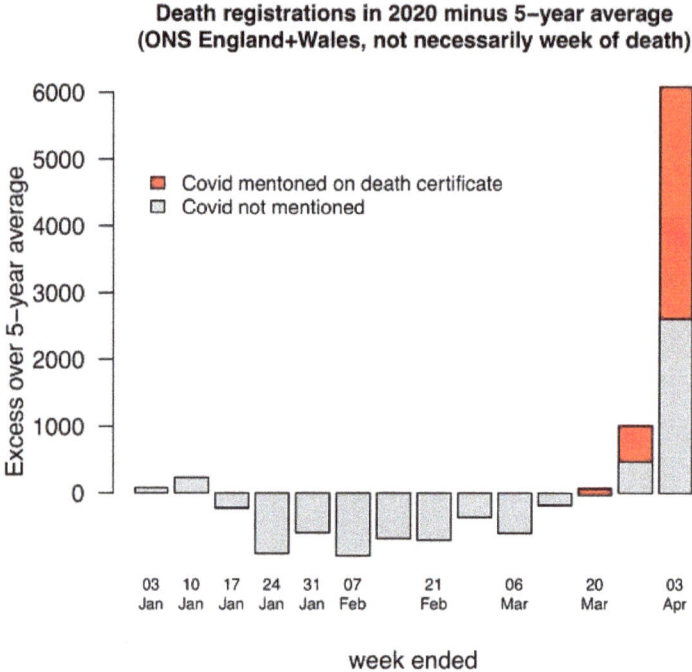

hardly trust government stats any more. As soon as people began discussing the anomalously low mortality for the first months of this year, then right after that the weekly mortality started to zoom up. On that 3rd of April week, one-fifth of all the deaths are COVID-related: we'll allude to this syndrome henceforth as C19.

The ONS website brazenly stated, "From 31 March 2020 these figures also show the number of deaths involving corona virus (COVID-19), based on any mention of COVID-19 on the death certificate." Have these people no shame? Deaths shoot up on the graphs, as of course they would from this loose and inclusive criterion.

We've all heard how the C19 'illness' or 'disease' is associated with lung disease, as the flu normally is. But the ONS breakdown for April showed it to be just as much linked to heart disease, to

Alzheimer's disease and to diabetes. This rag-bag of pre-existing conditions does *not* show some mystery new disease, it just shows bad medical logic by doctors who seem no longer able to comprehend cause and effect.

The *UK Column* commented that the sudden increase in mortality shown by these figures was *due to* the lockdown effect. That is certainly the simplest inference here. ('The Imperial College Bill Gates Connection' 5.4.20 at 3 minutes)

The three weeks of total mortality data in England and Wales *after* the lockdown adds up to *forty percent more* than the total for the three weeks *before*. That's an extra *thirteen thousand* deaths. Does that sound like your government is protecting you? Or does it sound more as if locking up everyone is a way of *getting rid of* the elderly and the infirm? We were all supposed to be happy in the springtime, remember? Whereas this indicates that stress and depression is killing people off. Here, you can do the maths:

<u>Weekly Office of National Statistics data</u>

<u>Total deaths England & Wales</u>

28 Feb	6 Mar	13 Mar	20 Mar	27 Mar	3 Apr	10 Apr	17 Apr
10,618	10,895	11,019	10,645	11,141	16,387	18,516	22,351

1 week before / 1 week after => 5% more

2 weeks before / 2 weeks after => 27% more

3 weeks after / 3 weeks before => 41% more

4 weeks after / 4 weeks before => 58% more

Whatever it is, it keeps getting worse! And it's totally centred around the spring equinox ie the government's lockdown date, no such affect exists for any other date. Four weeks after compared to before gives twenty-five thousand more deaths, a more than fifty percent increase! If a lockdown were helping, would one not expect some decrease in mortality?

The Nightingale Hospital in East London was built in just nine days as a massive operation involving the military, and has space for four thousand patients. But, as of mid-April it was almost empty, having treated just 19 patients over the Easter weekend (*Mail*, 15th April). Is an epidemic really happening, outside of the BBC studios? Various of these 'Nightingale' hospitals have opened up and remain embarrassingly empty. NHS hospitals had four times more empty beds than normal. (HSJ.co.uk), and yes this is partly because other cases have been pushed out in anticipation of a vast surge of C19 cases, which never happened.

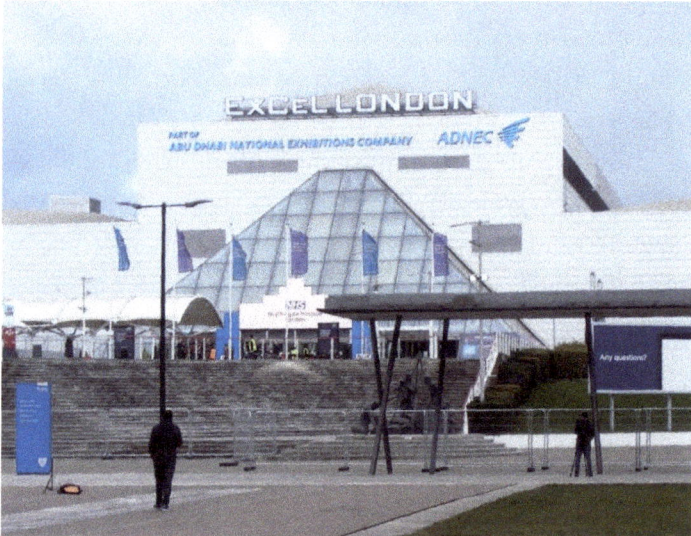

Figure: newly-built 'Nightingale' hospital in East London

Deaths trebled in care homes in England and Wales in a matter of weeks and why was that? The much-respected British historian David Starkey has described the startling events that took place over the spring equinox[5] in the NHS, immediately before the Lockdown:

> You stop all forms of surgery and diagnostic testing – completely. Cancer, heart disease – the lot. The NHS becomes

---

5 Starkey, 'Covid-19 -- Britain's Disastrous Response Will Have Devastating Consequences' 16 May at 13 mins

the National Covid Service. Secondly, you clear every bed that you can, to deal with the expected influx of Covid patients. This is when of course patients usually elderly who may well have had COVID-19 get sent back to care homes... a series of astonishing decisions ... a terrible price to pay, because we have got two other sets of deaths which are now catching up, there are the deaths of people who should have been treated for cancer and who should have been treated for heart disease, who are also terrified to go to hospital because of COVID-19, and therefore are dying in droves.. and there is the final sting in the tail that as deaths go down in hospitals they go up in care homes.

That goes a long way towards explain the shocking increase in old peoples' deaths following the Lockdown, Dr Starkey being one of the more respected intellectuals in the UK. In his view, 'a calamitous series of events and decisions caused a panicked British government to recklessly abandon its sensible coronavirus plan for one that is likely to harm the nation far more than the virus itself.' It would be hard to disagree with that. He described what has happened as 'a bizarre and unprecedented abandoning of the Hippocratic oath' which I think is a good phrase.

By the end of May there had been well over fifty thousand excess deaths in England and Wales, i.e. above the normal average values, since the lockdown began (ONS data). Compare that with the deficit of four thousand deaths for the same period just before the lockdown. This book argues that such an excess is *not* due to any virus, but rather the lockdown policies of the Government.

Here are a couple of nurses' comments, on blog sites: 'My fear is that the gov will agree to an endless lockdown because they've scared everyone so much they're too terrified to ever leave the house.' And 'I can only speak for my hospital but colleagues in London all saying the same. It feels like a massive overreaction.'

Old people are being asked to sign 'DNR' forms, 'Do Not Resuscitate' which again hardly inspires confidence. One in three of UK patients who enter hospital for C19 never come out and well over half the people put onto ventilators in NHS hospitals die,[6] which may help to account for why people are scared of going to hospital.

6 Daily Mail 29 April 'One in every three coronavirus patients who go into hospital never come out.'

2

There is No Pandemic

The whole aim of practical politics is to keep the populace alarmed (and hence clamorous to be led to safety) by an endless series of hobgoblins, most of them imaginary — H.L. Mencken

One week after the government decision to lockdown Britain had been made, the former Supreme Court Judge Lord Jonathan Sumption was discussing the UK response to C19 on the BBC *World at One* show:

> The real question is, is this serious enough to warrant putting most of our population into house imprisonment, wrecking our economy for an indefinite period, destroying businesses that honest and hardworking people have taken years to build up, saddling future generations with debt, depression, stress, heart attacks, suicides and unbelievable distress inflicted on millions of people who are not especially vulnerable, and will suffer only mild symptoms or none at all?   (Quoted in Spiked, Peter Hitchens 30.3.20)

Initially, every news announcement of a CV 'death' was given in the form of so-and-so who tested positive for C19 has died, for example:

Covid-19 related death

Posted Friday, 20 March 2020 by William Jones

Louise Stead, the Chief Executive at Royal Surrey NHS Foundation Trust, said:

"Sadly, we can confirm that two of our patients who were being cared for at Royal Surrey County Hospital, and who had tested positive for COVID-19, have died.

The patients were aged 99 and 66 years old and both had underlying health conditions. Their families have been informed and our thoughts and condolences are with them at this difficult and distressing time."

That would then get reported in the news as, a C19 death or death *due to* C19. However there is no necessary causal connection between that diagnoses and the death.

David Icke gave a two-hour interview on *London Live* and it soon gained four million hits before it was deleted: Ofcom is now investigating *London Live* for having allowed that interview after some alleged complaints! That was the first time that *London Live* had had a video deleted from its channel. Youtube then got busy deleting other Icke interviews – plus it announced it would wipe any other videos that also falsely linked Covid-19 to 5G mobile networks. That's a relief! One wouldn't want people upset by allegations that the new worldwide 5G networks – untested for public safety – might be making people ill, if not indeed putting all life on Earth in gravest peril. The Icke interview alluded to 5G as an "electro-magnetic technologically generated soup of radiation toxicity."" Soon after that Icke's whole Facebook page was deleted: and we're here talking about the world's most popular speaker, whatever one may think of his views.

At 23 minutes of the interview he states 'Anyone who gets ill, for any reason .. even falling down the stairs, they now get tested for Covid 19 … they get lots of positives, and [whatever they're in hospital for] if they've tested positive for Covid19, when they die they are diagnosed as having died from COVID-19.'

That's the trick. That's how it's done. In a conversation about the topic I would recommend using this very simple point. Deaths are just being re-classified with little by way of any increase in mortality. Anyone entering hospital is 'tested' for C19. Thereby the 'epidemic' is created by the 'test'.

Icke gave the example of comedian Eddie Large who had long suffered from a heart condition. He went into hospital after a heart failure, and was diagnosed as Covid-19. Papers reported 'Eddie Large died in hospital after testing positive for COVID-19'. His family has been angrily protesting at this.

The cause-of-death decision therefore becomes very arbitrary, with recent World Health Organization guidelines instructing certifiers to record COVID-19 on death certificates in the absence of testing, including where the disease is only 'assumed to have caused, or contributed to' death.[7] Whether taking their cues from the WHO or not, many nations are recording deaths of suspected and probable COVID-19 cases as deaths due to COVID-19. This becomes a paper exercise where 'COVID-19' is written down if it is merely a 'suspected' or 'probable' cause of death. The WHO guideline states:

> A death due to COVID-19 is defined for surveillance purposes as a death resulting from a clinically compatible illness, in a probable or confirmed COVID-19 case, unless there is a clear alternative cause of death that cannot be related to COVID disease eg trauma.'

What diseases are thus 'clinically compatible'? Diabetes, heart trouble, Alzeimer's disease, you name it. There *is no coherent group of symptoms*, there does not exist here a discernable illness that 'causes' the death. This WHO definition *creates the pandemic*, or the illusion thereof. A terrifying new scourge *appears* to exist, and will do so as long as that WHO definition is adhered to. The world can recover from this 'dreadful scourge' collapsing all economies *only* by adjusting that WHO definition!

The coronavirus is an alleged virus which does *not* lead to a specific illness or disease. Thus 'COVID-19 has no unique

---

7 WHO 'Guidelines for Certification and Classification of COVID-19 as cause of death'

symptoms of its own...For context, most of the coronavirus deaths in Italy (88%), UK (91%) and USA (99.1%) involve other health conditions.'[8] This reminds one of the AIDS scam whereby a so-called 'Acquired Immuno-Deficiency Syndrome' included a cluster of some twenty different diseases, which were bracketed together on the grounds that the patient allegedly had developed a lowered resistance to getting them. That group of illnesses would vary from one continent to another, and its doubtful if there was ever an isolated 'HIV' (Human Immuno-deficient Virus – an absurd concept if ever there was one) isolated. The concept was highly profitable for the pharmaceutical companies involved and helped gays to avoid taking responsibility for how their multiple-partner lifestyle was shortening their lives. We're looking at something here which has a similar level of nonexistence.

A letter in the *Daily Telegraph* (30 April) expressed dismay at this totally fluid category of death - 'if doctors are attributing all deaths in care homes to COVID-19.'

The population have been sufficiently scared that they may not want restrictions lifted: Members of the public do not want the lockdown eased as they are 'very, very worried' about corona-virus, government ministers are advised, as they prepare to make a decision over

'Presumed Covid-19'

SIR – My mother died last week in a care home at the age of 98. When my brother registered her death, as expected, the cause given was "frailty due to old age", but he was surprised to see that the doctor certifying the death had added "presumed Covid-19", an inclusion that also shocked the home's manager.

The day before our mother died, my brother was allowed to sit with her for an hour. His temperature was checked before he was admitted, but there was no form of isolation and none of the home's staff were wearing personal protective equipment.

If doctors are attributing all deaths in care homes to Covid-19, it makes a nonsense of any statistics and does great reputational damage to both individual care homes and to the care industry as a whole.

Tony Parkinson
Christchurch, Dorset

---

8 'COVID REVISED: Are New WHO Guidelines Adding to the Death Toll?' 21st century Wire 19 April.

extending the lockdown next week**.'** (Mail 13 April 'Will terrified public leave lockdown even when they can?' Most people do NOT want restrictions lifted')

Is there a COVID-19 Virus?

Does it exist? Here is a medical expert view, probably as good sense on the matter as we're likely to get. 'PCR' is the name for the test developed by Kary Mullis in 1984 that doctors are using:

> Here's the problem, we are testing people for any strain of a Coronavirus. Not specifically for COVID-19. There are no reliable tests for a specific COVID-19 virus…This is why you're hearing that most people with COVID-19 are showing nothing more than cold/flu like symptoms. That's because most Coronavirus strains exhibit nothing more than cold/flu like symptoms. The few actual novel Coronavirus cases do have some worse respiratory responses, but still have a very promising recovery rate, especially for those without prior issues…The 'gold standard' in testing for COVID-19 would be laboratory isolated/purified coronavirus particles free from any contaminants and particles that look like viruses but are not, that have been proven to be the cause of the syndrome known as COVID-19 and obtained by using proper viral isolation methods and controls. PCR basically takes a sample of your cells and amplifies any DNA to look for 'viral sequences', i.e. bits of non-human DNA that seem to match parts of a known viral genome.
>
> The problem is the test is known not to work. It uses 'amplification' which means taking a very, very tiny amount of DNA and growing it exponentially until it can be analyzed. Obviously any minute contaminations in the sample will also be amplified leading to potentially gross errors of discovery. Additionally, it's only looking for partial viral sequences, not

whole genomes, so identifying a single pathogen is next to impossible even if you ignore the other issues.

The Mickey Mouse test kits being sent out to hospitals, at best, tell analysts you have some viral DNA in your cells. Which most of us do, most of the time. It may tell you the viral sequence is related to a specific type of virus – say the huge family of coronavirus. But that's all. The idea these kits can isolate a specific virus like COVID-19 is nonsense.

If you feel sick and get a PCR test any random virus DNA might be identified even if they aren't at all involved in your sickness which leads to false diagnosis.

And coronavirus are incredibly common. A large percentage of the world population will have covi DNA in them in small quantities even if they are perfectly well, or indeed sick with some other pathogen.

Do you see where this is going yet? If you want to create a totally false panic about a totally false pandemic – pick a coronavirus.

They are incredibly common and there's tons of them. A very high percentage of people who have become sick by other means (flu, bacterial pneumonia or almost anything) will have a positive PCR test for covi even if you're doing them properly and ruling out contamination, simply because covis are so common.

There are hundreds of thousands of flu and pneumonia victims in hospitals throughout the world at any one time. All you need to do is select the sickest of these in a single location – say Wuhan – administer PCR tests to them and claim anyone showing viral sequences similar to a coronavirus (which will inevitably be quite a few) is suffering from a 'new' disease. Since you already selected the sickest flu cases a fairly high proportion of your sample will go on to die.

You can then say this 'new' virus has a CFR higher than the flu and use this to infuse more concern and do more tests which will of course produce more 'cases', which expands the testing, which produces yet more 'cases' and so on and so on.[9]

Was that what really happened, was it all just bad logic and bogus theory? Fear is the drug, it's what the public need. There is a problem that 'due to the fact there is no actual new deadly pathogen but just regular sick people' people will sooner or later notice there's no increase in deaths. And so,

1. You can claim this is just the beginning and more deaths are imminent. Use this as an excuse to quarantine everyone and then claim the quarantine prevented the expected millions of dead.
2. You can tell people that 'minimizing' the dangers is irresponsible and bully them into not talking about numbers.

Here is a shorter (and satirical) comment from John Rappaport, one of the few people who do seem to understand the biochemistry: "Sir, I want to tell you that the inherently worthless PCR we just ran on you was also contaminated with who knows how many meaningless germs, and there is a hundred percent chance that, when I tell you now you are a coronavirus case, I haven't the slightest idea in the world what I'm talking about. However, we are going to hospitalize you and give you very toxic and dangerous antiviral drugs."

That'll do, we've got the picture. The fix is in.

Percent mortality in CV+ Cases

The World Health Organization has stated, 'Coronavirus is ten times deadlier than the 2009 swine flu pandemic and a vaccine will be needed to halt it… As a percentage, coronavirus has so far killed

---

9 *Global Research,* Julian Rose 27 March 'Manufactured Pandemic: Testing People for Any Strain of a Coronavirus, Not Specifically for COVID-19'

6.4 per cent of people who have tested positive for it, including 12 per cent of those in Britain, 0.1 per cent in Australia and 4 per cent in the US.' (*The Mail* 14 April 'coronavirus is ten times deadlier than the 2009 swine flu epidemic, WHO reveals') That totally unhinged judgement led swiftly to calls for a mandatory vaccine.

The solution turned out to be for the WHO to acknowledge that 'ultimately, the development and delivery of a safe and effective vaccine will be needed to fully interrupt transmission.' Any 'vaccine' liable to be developed, will be those which tamper with your DNA – not something ever allowed before. That is what we may call the Bill Gates solution, where the 'vaccine' will adjust your DNA – putting the future of the human race at risk! Soon you may not be able to get an air flight, or a lot of other things, unless you have the vaccine…

That WHO lethality estimate was far too high and that high estimate was a central part of the original fear message. Let us ask, what proportion of a CV+ sampled population may be expected to die? An independent Swiss group calling itself Swiss Propaganda Research found that 60% to 80% of people who test positive remain symptom-free, that even among over-seventies, 60% of those who test positive are free of symptoms, and many others have only very mild symptoms. It gave a crucially important judgment about lethality, ie what % of those who test positive then die – and it's only a few tenths of one percent:

> According to data from the best-studied countries such as South Korea, Iceland and Germany as well as the cruise ship *Diamond Princess*, the overall lethality of Covid19 is in the *per mille*[10] range and thus about ten times lower than initially assumed by the WHO.

10 Per mille => parts per thousand

A study in *Nature Medicine* comes to a similar conclusion even for the Chinese city of Wuhan. The initially significantly higher values for Wuhan were obtained because many people with mild or no symptoms were not recorded.[11]

A comparable study was reported in *The Economist,* using US data: 'Silverman and Washburne found that the coronavirus mortality rate could be as low as 0.1 percent, similar to that of flu.'[12] The idea here is that "If millions of people were infected weeks ago without dying, the virus must be less deadly than official data suggest." Clearly if the mortality is anything like as low as one or two parts per thousand, then it is no higher than the flu and the optimal policy would have been to do nothing, or to rephrase that we'd have been better off if no-one had ever 'invented' CV-19. Far higher estimates were obtained initially by sampling sick people and those going into hospital.

And the study[13] at Stanford University in California was by Dr. John Ioannidis, regarded as one of the most trustworthy US medical authorities. He took blood samples from a population of Santa Clara County in California and based on that they estimated the C19 mortality rate at 0.14% or less, meaning 14 deaths or fewer per 10,000 people infected. Worldwide, that would imply that millions were likely to have been infected with the novel coronavirus, and its lethality would be about the same as that of the seasonal flu. Researchers found Covid-19 antibodies in those not admitted to hospital and inferred that the true number of cases exceeded official records by 50-85 times, with most suffering mild or no symptoms.

---

11 *Nature Medicine* volume 26, pages506–510(2020) 'Estimating clinical severity of COVID-19 from the transmission dynamics in Wuhan, China' Joseph T. Wu *et al.* (9 authors)
12 *The Economist* 11 April, 'Why a study showing that COVID 19 is everywhere is good news'
13 April 17th, 'COVID-19 Antibody Seroprevalence in Santa Clara County, California' published in MedRxiv

Dr Ioannidis can be watched explaining this investigation ('Perspectives on the Pandemic' 19 April), and how he found out how many people in Santa Clara had encountered the CV virus, by investigating the 'antibodies' formed. The lower 'infection fatality rate' was 'in the same ball-park' as seasonal flu.

Age-specific mortality rates due to COVID-19, per 100,000 people, England and Wales, occurring in March 2020

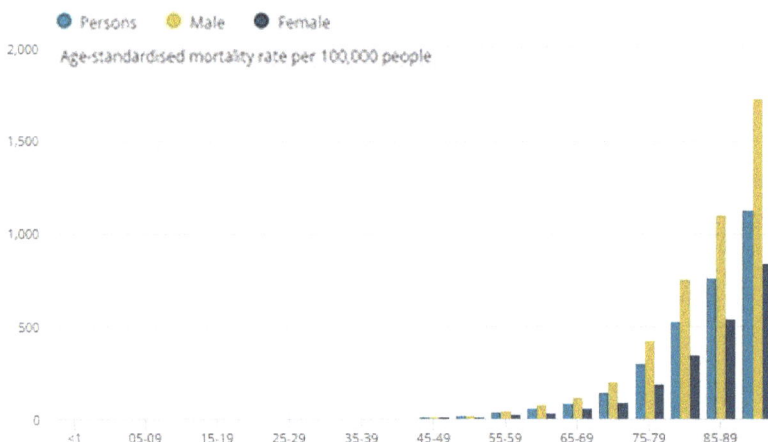

Source: Office for National Statistics – Analysis of deaths involving COVID-

It's the old folk who die. Half of all the people in Europe who 'died of coronavirus' were in old people's homes, according to the World Health Organization,[14] the WHO European director describing this as an 'unimaginable human tragedy.' Far from being unimaginable it was totally predictable and in fact many had predicated it: old people die *because* they are isolated, and isolation causes them to give up hope. An ONS mortality graph for April here shows age distribution.[15] The average age of people diagnosed as

14 Mail 'Nearly half of all European coronavirus cases were care home residents' April 24.
15ons.gov.uk/peoplepopulationandcommunity/birthsdeathsandmarruiages/deaths 'Deaths involving COVID-19'

dying from C19, is generally over eighty!

Question: What kind of illness targets mainly very old people?

Answer: a bogus illness that can be linked to persons about to die off anyhow.

That graph shows that it is *not* a real illness or disease: what it does show is exactly what David Icke said was going on, viz that anyone entering a hospital is being tested for C19, so old people likely to die thus 'test positive.' Children are immune from getting 'it' as the graph clearly shows. Schoolchildren are being stressed-out and probably quite psychologically damaged by the social distancing so they cannot play and can hardly go to school. They have a gun-like instrument pointed at their head to measure temperature. And all for what?

The Peak of Infection?

The '21st Century Wire' site of Patrick Hennigan has been calling out the monster hoax which caused the UK lockdown:

> Moreover, we have consistently stated across many media platforms that these were not science-based decisions either, but rather political decisions taken by government officials as part of a mass-panic, alongside a parallel roll-out of a broader authoritarian agenda. For this, our publication and its contributors were attacked and marginalised by other media outlets and pundits who insisted this was a 'conspiracy theory' and that we should accept the government's rationale for unprecedented lockdown policies and the suspension of democracy and civil liberties. However, since then, a number of eminent experts have emerged who are also saying the same thing we were over the duration of this crisis.

It quoted the Oxford University 'Centre for evidence-Based Medecine' as stating that the peak of the 'crisis' actually came a full week before Boris Johnson initiated lockdown on March 23rd, on the grounds that infection happens some three weeks before. In an interview with the Mail Online the professor Dr Heneghan explained:

> The peak of deaths occurred on April 8, and if you understand that then you work backwards to find the peak of infections. That would be 21 days before then, right before the point of lockdown.

Number of people who died with coronavirus in hospital each day

Here is a graph from a BBC website, showing NHS daily data.[16] It illustrates the Oxford unit's claim that a peak occurred on April 8th. This data implies a timespan of the outbreak comparable to seasonal flu., as well as the peak of infection being some three weeks earlier. We'll see how stats from a month later will slightly adjust that peak to April 11th, but the logic here remains perfectly sound.

Politicians talk a lot about 'flattening the curve,' as in, 'We hope that the curve is flattening now', when they claim to be 'following the science.' Well the curve flattened on April 11th and it's been going down since then. Men are more likely to get 'it'.

---

16 BBC News, 'Coronavirus: Deaths at 20-year high but peak may be over' 21 April

Lockdown or not? Comparing the nations

Dr Heneghan admired the way Sweden had managed to resist the panic:

> Some of the non-lockdown states like Sweden have done well to 'hold their nerve' while eschewing popular 'doomsday scenarios' which were being pushed incessantly by governments and media in order to justify draconian lockdown policies. The Scandinavian country has recorded just 392 new patients and 40 deaths today [19th April], approximately 10 per cent of the UK totals.

Here is a graph showing total deaths cumulatively (per million) of Sweden and the UK, as prepared by John Hopkins University. It goes up to 19th April, 2000.

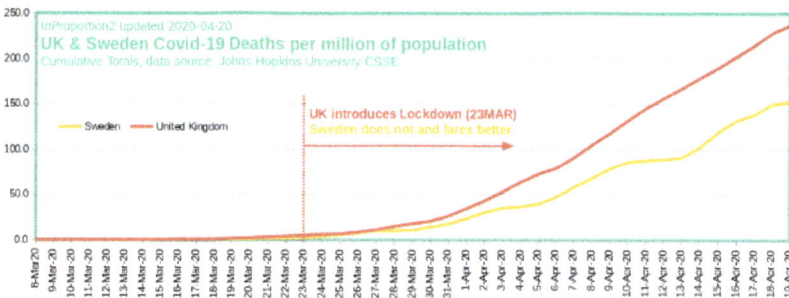

Figure: Sweden (yellow line) and UK (red line) compared, of daily C19 deaths per million, showing the date of 23rd March when lockdown began.

Or, we could make a more general comparison of European nations. To do this we count the total C19-diagnosed deaths and express these per million of population. For March 1st, 2021 the UK then had an almost-top position in Europe for reported C19 deaths:[17]

---

17 Using the 'worldometer' site, eg worldometers.info/coronavirus/country/france

National totals of 'C19 deaths' up to 1.3.21, per million

Belgium 1936   UK   1851   Italy 1624 USA 1607 Spain 1484
France   1296   Sweden 1276 Germany 854   Israel   643

Within Europe, Sweden which did not impose the lockdown would appear to have a lower incidence than other countries except for Germany. Here is a graph prepared by *UK Column* showing CV deaths per million,[18] with 'lockdown countries' in red versus non-lockdown in Green. The figures aren't quite the same as above and would have been obtained a few days earlier.

Figure: non-lockdown countries in green (Sweden, Iceland, Belarus, Taiwan, S. Korea, Japan & Mexico) compared to lockdown countries in red (UK, France, Germany, Spain, Italy, Belgium & USA). Mexico did later impose a lockdown.

In Britain, one person in three thousand had died after testing positive with coronavirus and for the USA the corresponding figure was one person in six thousand: was that really worth a nationwide lockdown?

---

18 From Vanessa Beeley UKColumn article 'Who controls British government response to covid19'

On the same day as this bar-chart was compiled by *UK Column*, an Oxford University project published a study of what they called 'stringency' of lockdown for different nations, comparing it to their C19 mortality. Here is their graph[19], and it showed a positive correlation, ie the more the lockdown the greater the incidence of 'coronavirus' mortality.

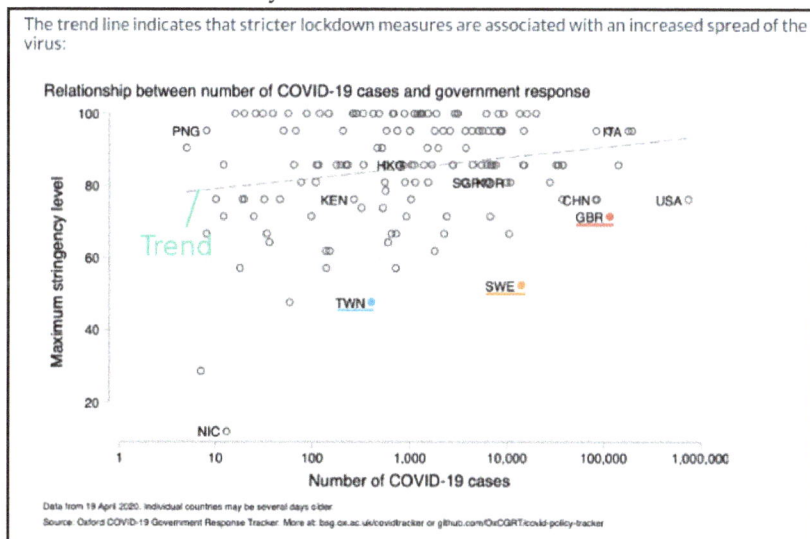

The trend line indicates that stricter lockdown measures are associated with an increased spread of the virus:

Relationship between number of COVID-19 cases and government response

Data from 19 April 2020. Individual countries may be several days older

Source: Oxford COVID-19 Government Response Tracker. More at: bsg.ox.ac.uk/covidtracker or github.com/OxCGRT/covid-policy-tracker

Figure: The graph plots different countries by 'Stringency level' (vertical axis) and their number of C19 cases (horizontal axis). A best-fit straight line through the data, shows the former increase with the latter. Source: Oxford C19 Govt. Response Tracker.

This is a result that should have made newspaper headlines around the world. The first ever truly global experiment, in which all countries participated, Northern and Southern hemispheres alike – and the results are in! But the Oxford team only allowed themselves the rather cautious comment seen at the top of this graph. Presumably they'd be in hot water had they publicly announced this result.

---

19 bsg.ox.ac.uk/covidtracker This graph for May 18th is an updated version of their month-earlier original.

A comment upon this result did appear ten days later, by a Mr Iain Davies writing in the *Off-Guardian*: 'Nor is there any evidence that lockdown regimes have any positive impact upon infections rates. Comparisons between severe lockdown states and those who opted for less draconian measures reveal no advantage to placing your population under house arrest... Oxford University found *a direct correlation between infection rates and the relative severity of lockdown regimes. It suggests the more stringent the lockdown, the higher the infection rate.* This is not unexpected, as numerous epidemiological studies have shown that infection rates for C19 are higher when people are exposed to it for prolonged periods in confined spaces. Locking people up in their homes is probably the worst thing you could do if you wanted to reduce the infections and the duration of the outbreak.'[20]

That is really the most important conclusion, and it is gratifying to have had two independent sources confirm the same result. No notice was taken by the British media.

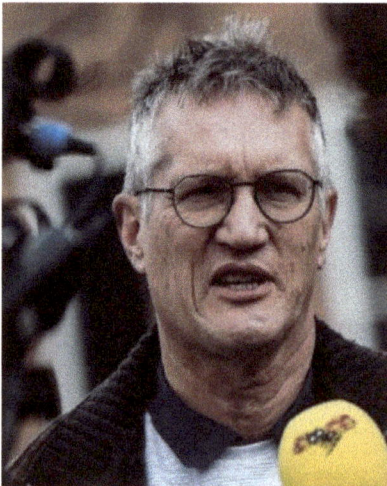

Sweden has persevered in its sensible no-lockdown policy, and Mr Anders Tegnell, its chief epidemiologist, has become something of a hero, with people tattooing his image on their arms! Yes its rate has been higher than for neighbouring nations such as

Figure: Swedish no-lockdown hero Anders Tegnell.

Norway and Denmark, *however* Sweden has no fear of a

---

20 off-guardian.org/2020/04/29/lokin-20-the-lockdown-regime-causes-increasing-health-concerns/

'second wave' later arriving, as other European nations do have. [21]

Britain comes Top!

On May 4th ('May the fourth be with you') the UK surged ahead in terms of total CV 'deaths' overtaking Spain and Italy. That meant that the US and UK were leading the world in this respect. In terms of deaths per million, the UK was way above France, Italy, Spain and the USA. Was this a consequence of a further loosening up of the definition announced in mid-April? The state had already given the incredibly vague advice that:

> If before death the patient had symptoms typical of COVID 19 infection....it would be satisfactory to give 'COVID-19' as the cause of death.[22]

Then on 14th of April the criteria became even vaguer:

> From this week, the death notifications we collect from providers will allow them to report whether the death was of a person with suspected or confirmed Covid-19.[23]

That was from a spokesperson of the 'Care Quality Commission,' whatever that is. Thus, the 'provider' need not be medically qualified and can report a C19-death if 'typical' symptoms are reported or if the person was 'suspected' to be C19-positive. This data is then added onto the claimed C19 mortality figures. Why, there was not even a need for a PCR test to certify such a death:

> A doctor can certify the involvement of COVID-19 based on symptoms and clinical findings – a positive test resul is

---

21 rt.com/news/488968-sweden-model-excessive-deaths/
22 ONS, Guidance for doctors Completing Medical Certificates, 3.
23 For refs see https://off-guardian.org/2020/04/29/lokin-20-the-lockdown-regime-causes-increasing-health-concerns/

not required.[24]

But the condition hardly had symptoms, or no distinctive symptoms - that was the problem. Dr John Lee in the *Spectator* well expressed this paradox:[25]

> The majority of cases are asymptomatic. The most common symptoms are not fever, cough, headache and respiratory symptoms; they are no symptoms at all. The typical case does not suffer respiratory fibrosis; the disease leaves no mark. Somewhere around 99.9 per cent of those who catch the disease recover. Of those unlucky enough to die, over 90 per cent have pre-existing conditions and were anyway approaching the end of their lives.

There is no proper concept of causality here: how can people take seriously so woolly a procedure with its phantomic 'cause of death' concept? If we're being told that a virus called 'SARS-CoV-2' causes the illness 'COVID-19', that sounds a lot like linguistic trickery. Here one can only quote the ironic judgment of Iain Davies: 'C19 is the first disease in history from which you can officially die without any firm evidence that you actually had it.' (From his brilliant *Off-Guardian* article, reference 23, above)

On that dramatic May 4th, as news of Britain coming top of the league was announced, journalists were not required to exercise their judgment on this matter, because a juicy sex-scandal hit the headlines – well-timed no doubt. Neil Ferguson was being relieved of his position, on account of an extra-marital affair he'd been having: he broke 'social distancing rules.' He had become a liability on account of increasing public awareness of his appalling track record with hugely exaggerated death-predictions – generally speaking a couple of hundred times too high, as we see in a later chapter. But even then they would not sack him and he was allowed

---

24 ONS 'Deaths Registered Weekly in England & wales, 9 Glossary.
25 John Lee, The Spectator, 8 May, 'Ten Reasons to End the Lockdown Now'

to resign.

What we may wonder is the meaning of the two most warlike of nations, the US and UK, always claiming to have a special relationship, getting to this top position? Whereas Russia has fewer deaths in proportion than any other northern-hemisphere country, at around 10 per million. It's estimated that 80% of the C19 dead have been in NATO nations, with the highest death per million being in Belgium, NATO HQ. It would take a brave man to comment upon this!

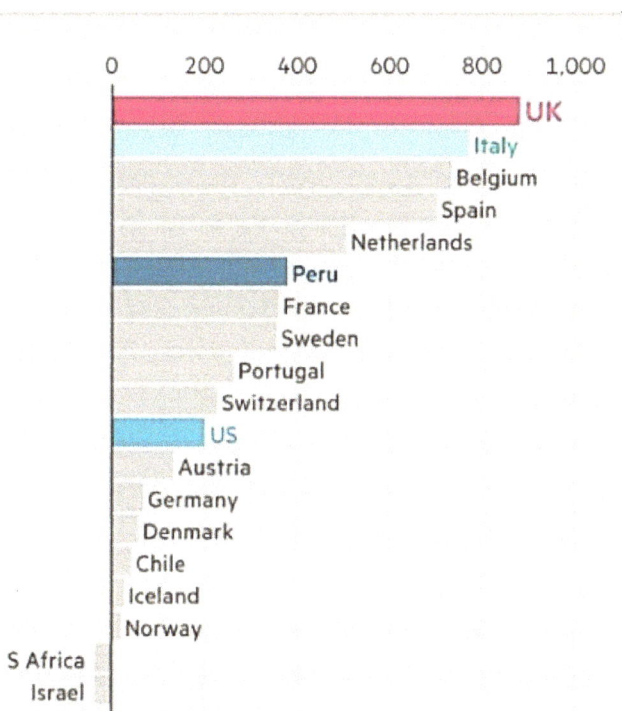

Figure: *Financial Times* analysis showing total Excess-deaths-since-pandemic-began per million of population, 28 May. UK is top, Italy second and Belgium third.

US hospitals are paid *pro rata* for their C19 cases. They receive $13,000 per Covid-19 admission, plus also there's an extra $39,000 if those patients receive ventilator treatment, which must push up the numbers quite a bit.

At the end of May, Britain was described as the top of *all nations* for coronavirus deaths! This analysis came from the *Financial Times,* which concluded 'The UK has suffered the highest rate of deaths from the coronavirus pandemic among countries that produce comparable data.' They reported this (on 28 May) because 'the level of excess deaths in other hard-hit European countries, such as Italy and Spain, has returned close to normal levels.' They had counted all 'excess deaths' recorded, ie above average levels, since the pandemic began. Thus it was not merely deaths attributed to Coronavirus they were counting, but rather what Chapter 1 called 'total mortality,' and that in excess above the average for previous years.

The title of this FT article, 'UK suffers highest death rate from coronavirus' is however misleading: these deaths are not 'from coronavirus' but are a *consequence of* the lockdown and result from the enormous stress and distress which people are experiencing especially in care homes for the elderly. Thus a *British Medical journal* concluded 'Only a third of the excess deaths seen in the community in England and Wales can be explained by Covid-19.'[26] It described how this huge number of unexplained deaths has been alluded to by the chair of Centre for Risk and Evidence Communication at the University of Cambridge, on May 12th: over the past five weeks he said, care homes and other community settings had to deal with a 'staggering burden' of 30,000 more deaths than would normally be expected. He added, 'When we look back . . . this rise in non-covid extra deaths outside the hospital is something I hope will be given really severe attention.' That surge in deaths - which promoted the UK to the unenviable number one position of alleged-C19 deaths worldwide - indicates the catastrophic error that has been made. One GP who had to sign the death certificates has concluded quite

---

[26] Bmj.com '"Staggering number" of extra deaths in community is not explained by covid-19,' Shaun Griffin, 13.5.20.

rightly that 'If ... lockdown killed the other 30,000, then the lockdown was a complete and utter waste of time and should never happen again.'[27]

Consider the following about coronavirus (or, 'SARs-CoV-2' as it is known) from the Swiss Policy Research group (See appendix 1)[28]

> The median age of the deceased in most countries (including Italy) is <u>over 80 years</u> (e.g. 86 years in Sweden) and <u>only about 4%</u> of the deceased had no serious preconditions. The age and risk profile of deaths thus essentially corresponds to normal mortality.

Medical professionals can surely benefit from consulting the Swiss policy research conclusions, of which this is one. In their view, 4% of 'C19 deaths' are not caused by old age or heart attacks or lung infections etc. but may specifically be a result of the COVID virus. The average value of the seven European nations in the above table is 550, or one person in 1800 dying. Taking 4% of that as the deaths that were 'really' due to the Coronavirus and not other factors, that will gives us one 'real' COVID death per fifty thousand people; which, over six months, is not very much.

The Act

The British lockdown synchronized, oddly enough, with the 'Coronavirus Act' passed on 'lockdown day' March 23rd. Outrageous powers of arrest were given to the police, and there was no requirement for post-mortems for any 'coronavirus death' – which many felt was a vital part of the monster hoax. Excerpts:

41 (1) Compliance with a direction issued under this Part of this Schedule may be enforced by — (a) a constable; (b) any other person, or description of person, designated in writing for the purpose of this

---

[27] Malcolm Kendrick, 'I've signed death certificates during Covid-19. Here's why you can't trust any of the statistics on the number of victims' rt.com 28 May.
[28] https://swprs.org/a-swiss-doctor-on-covid-19/

paragraph by the Executive Office. (2)

In exercising the power of enforcement conferred by sub-paragraph (1), a person may— (a) enter any premises; (b) if necessary, use reasonable force.

This means the government can appoint anyone they like to come round your house, force entry and haul you away. "Description of a person" means any gang the named person decides to take along with him/her.

Offences 42 (1) A person commits an offence if the person fails without reasonable excuse to comply with a prohibition, requirement or restriction imposed on the person by a direction issued under this Part of this Schedule.

(2) A person guilty of an offence under this paragraph is liable—

(a) on summary conviction, to a fine not exceeding £100,000;

(b) on conviction on indictment, to a fine.

We're not even told who has to give the prohibition (No, Ma'am you can't walk your dog). The magnitude of the possible fine means in effect that 'they' have the power to confiscate your home if you do not obey.

Applications for compulsory admission to hospital for assessment or treatment (p.90)

3 (1) An application by an approved mental health professional under section 2 or 3 made during a period for which this paragraph has effect may be founded on a recommendation by a single registered medical practitioner (a "single recommendation"), if the professional considers that compliance with the requirement under that section for the recommendations of two practitioners is impractical or would involve undesirable delay

Page 91 (Period of remand to hospital)

5 Sections 35(7) (period of remand to hospital for report on mental condition) and 36(6) (period of remand to hospital for treatment) have effect as if the words "or for more than 12 weeks in all" were omitted.

This means that *one person's opinion* (with no second opinion required) can get you locked up in a mental health facility. In the past the Mental Health Act (1983) has always required two or three people to co-sign for a person to be put away, and having just one single 'mental health practitioner' able to do that is very disturbing. You can be suddenly removed, in theory to just about anywhere, if someone *suspects* that you *might be* infectious:

Powers relating to potentially Infectious Persons in England(p.217):

Powers to direct or remove persons to a place suitable for screening and assessment 6 (1) This paragraph applies if, during a transmission control period, a public health officer has reasonable grounds to suspect that a person in England is potentially infectious.

2) The public health officer may, subject to sub-paragraph (3) (a) direct the person to go immediately to a place specified in the direction which is suitable for screening and assessment, (b) remove the person to a place suitable for screening and assessment, or (c) request a constable to remove the person to a place suitable for screening and assessment (and the constable may then do so).

These words carry a potential for 'totalitarian abuse' that the state has granted itself, where the individual has no recourse or redress. This applies if somebody *suspects* that you *might* be infectious. With these new powers a 'public health officer' (whatever that is) can do just about anything they want.

Page 221: (2) A public health officer may at any time during the transmission control period impose such requirements and restrictions on the person as the officer considers necessary and proportionate—

(a) in the interests of the person,

b) for the protection of other people, or

(c) for the maintenance of public health.

(3) Requirements under this paragraph may include requirements—

(a) to provide information to the public health officer or any specified person;

(b) to provide details by which the person may be contacted during a specified period; (c) to go for the purposes of further screening and assessment to a specified place suitable for those purposes and do anything that may be required under paragraph 10(1);

(d) to remain at a specified place (which may be a place suitable for screening and assessment) for a specified period;

(e) to remain at a specified place in isolation from others for a specified period.

So a bureaucrat or 'health official' can tell you to go to 'a specified place' and remain there for 'a specified time' – alone! This new Act is a lot more frightening than any virus. An important section involves the test and death certificate.

Page 129, Signing of certificates of cause of death, 23 (1). This paragraph applies if— (a) a person dies as a result of any natural illness, (b) the person was treated by a registered medical practitioner ("A") within 28 days prior to the date of the person's death, (c) the time when (apart from this paragraph) A would be required to sign the certificate of cause of death under Article 25(2) falls within any period for which this paragraph has effect, (d) at that time, A is unable to sign the certificate or it is impracticable for A to do so, and (e) another registered medical practitioner ("B") can state to the best of B's knowledge and belief the cause of death. (2) B may sign the certificate of cause of death under Article 25(2). (3) B is subject to the other duties applicable to a person who has signed such a certificate. (4) A is not subject to any duties in relation to such a certificate. 24 (1) This paragraph applies if—

(a) a person dies as a result of any natural illness,

(b) the person was not treated by a registered medical practitioner within 28 days prior to the date of the person's death, and

(c) a registered medical practitioner ("C") can state to the best of C's knowledge and belief the cause of death. (2) C may sign the certificate of cause of death under Article 25(2). (3) C is subject to the other duties applicable to a person who has signed such a certificate. 25 Where B or C proposes to sign a certificate under Article 25(2) in reliance on paragraph 23 or 24, Form 12 has effect as if— (a) the two lines beginning with "Date on which was last seen alive and treated by me" were omitted …

Thus responsibility for reporting accurately on a cause of death has slipped from 'person A' (a doctor who attended the patient prior to that patient's death) to persons "B" and even "C". Thereby doctors can evade taking responsibility for statements about the deaths of patients they have treated and facilitates the statistical manipulation of the deaths. One begins to sense *how the trick is done* to generate the illusion of a pandemic.

This 358-page Coronavirus Act must have taken *at least* a month to prepare. It was passed by Parliament on 23rd March without a vote, then two days later zoomed thru the House of Lords and gained Royal Assent! Described as "the most extensive encroachment on British civil liberties … ever seen outside of wartime,"[29] the Act clearly violates a whole lot of *Magna Carta* principles on which British justice had hitherto been based.

There had been no time for a parliamentary debate: "By reason of urgency, it is necessary to make this instrument without a draft having been laid before, and approved by, a resolution of, each

29 Dunt, Ian 18.3.20 "Coronavirus bill: The biggest expansion in executive power we've seen in our lifetime". Politics.co.uk.

House of Parliament." We've heard that one before.

This Act reminds one of the US Patriot Act passed a week after the 9/11 event, which was very detailed and had clearly been prepared a long time in advance, and greatly abrogated the US constitution. By its very detail it showed that the event had been meticulously planned.

3

Advance Planning

> ...advanced forms of biological warfare that can 'target' specific genotypes may transform biological warfare from the realm of terror to a politically useful tool.
>
> Pentagon document 2000 'Rebuilding America's Defences,' p.60

Such a major global event needs proper advance planning. We could here start in late 2017, when Dr Anthony Fauci, the US Government's "pandemic advisor" and head of the National Institute of Allergy and Infectious Diseases, gave a speech on 'Pandemic Preparedness in the Next Administration' days before Trump was inaugurated. He averred:

> There is no question that there will be a challenge to the coming administration in the arena of infectious diseases...
> But also there will be a surprise outbreak.

How did he know that? Under the Obama administration Fauci had been in charge of the National Institute for Heath and in 2015 it transferred $3.7 million to a Wuhan virus-related laboratory. A moratorium had been placed upon coronavirus research and this seems to have been a way of getting around that prohibition.

Wuhan with its eleven million inhabitants is very much at the centre of China, and sits on the junction of the Han river and the Yangzi. Twenty miles outside it, the high-level bioweapon lab was constructed just two years before the C19 struck.

On August 13th, 2019 a four-day *Operation Crimson Contagion* was held in Washington DC. It planned for a 'global influenza pandemic' which featured school closures, social distancing, medical countermeasures etc. with everyone being told to stay at home. Its *Pandemic Crisis Action Plan* had been prepared earlier, in January.

Nineteen federal agencies participated, and its storyline had visitors from China who inadvertently carried the new virus into the USA. It was co-organized by a Disaster Leadership Group and an NSC Domestic Resilience Group.

One commentator observed here that '*The fake flu pandemic eerily mirrors the real coronavirus outbreak the U.S. is struggling with now*' (govtech.com Emergency Management, 20.3.20). It did not 'eerily mirror' the event, it was a blueprint for it.

A few months after that the Event 201 was held in October 2019, a 'Global Pandemic Exercise' was organized by the Bill and Melinda Gates Foundation with the World Economic Forum and the Michael Bloomberg School of Public Health. Held at the Johns Hopkins University's Center for Health Security, it simulated a global coronavirus outbreak. Its brochure began with the firm statement: 'We need to prepare for the event that becomes a pandemic.' It imagined a new form of coronavirus as developing from bats to pigs to farmers. The infected people develop a respiratory illness with symptoms ranging from mild, flu-like signs to severe pneumonia. The virus is able to travel through the air – which N.B., no virus can do - and 'unless it is quickly controlled' it could lead to a severe worldwide pandemic, 'an outbreak that circles the globe.' The Irish doctor Michael Ryan told the Event 201 team that: I fully expect that we will be confronted by a fast-moving highly lethal pandemic of a respiratory pathogen.'

A Pandemic Emergency Board *has been set up* [the tone was that of a normal news announcement in the past tense], a spokesman from the John Hopkins Center for Health Security' explained. The event was deliberately using the format of a news program in order to clothe themselves with some semblance of credibility. An *exponential increase* was predicted for the new threat and it could *only be resolved* by global business and governments working together. 'Pandemic anti-virals' have to be produced and distributed. A 'UN

Foundation' lady discusses how the countries most affected *have been* the lower-income ones. Flights are cancelled, and we're all advised: do not travel, stay at home! The pandemic leads to a 15% collapse of global financial markets. The head of the Chinese CDC

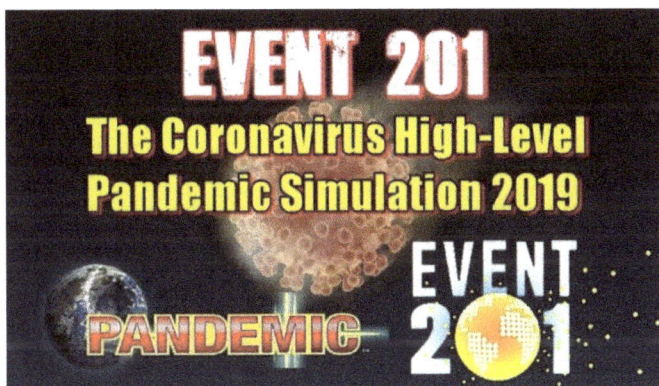

was present, and what was he doing there?

The conference developed the 'trusted voice' concept: of finding in each country who was regarded as trustworthy – to promote their awful new fiction![30] Persons around the table spoke of how important it was to find those voices. 'Do we need to find them now, and establish trust in those voices now?' Neil Ferguson was presumably the 'trusted voice' for the UK! '… so that when the crisis hits, people would already have the established trust.' One notes the 'when,' not 'if:' the crisis *is going to* hit and the built-up 'trust' has to be there *before* it happens. It was necessary to 'identify the community and faith-based leaders in particular' – would they be more trusting? Alarming pictures of empty shelves in shops were shown. As to their audience, 'The Board's recommendations are aimed at top decision-makers in national governments.' Another member spoke of how important it was to delete and prevent

---

[30] See Richplanet.net show 282 'Exposing the Man behind the Corona Virus scam' at 22 minutes.

'misinformation' from social media – i.e., views sceptical of the monster hoax they were about to perpetrate.

The John Hopkins University kept the 'numbers' of the game-simulation played out through the table-top exercise 'Event 201' that was run under the 'World Economic Forum,' six weeks before the actual CV outbreak was first reported.. It also keeps all of the real-world numbers, i.e. the graphs with red spots on them, continually updated, etc.

That event was a detailed blueprint of what then happened six weeks later. As Bill Gates made his fortune by selling Microsoft all around the world, so now a vaccine is going to be developed and sold, all around Planet Earth. He has of course no medical qualifications whatsoever.

These were the two major US desktop game-simulations which led up to the actual event. These comprise the steps of imagining and blueprinting the event, *which then happens. The event therefore originates within the US.* We are reminded here of Webster Tarpley's dictum,

> No terrorist attack would be complete without the advance airing of a scenario docudrama to provide the population with a conceptual scheme to help them understand the coming events in the sense intended by the oligarchy (Synthetic Terror, 2004, p.408).

Those who have studied the London Bombing of July 2005 will be aware of a *Panorama* program in May of 2004, fairly exactly describing what was going to happen, and using just the same tone of a scenario docudrama as in the 'Event 201' *as if* the news were being reported.

US Intelligence knew of the emerging coronavirus outbreak in China as early as mid-November, because it then gave Israel an advance warning, an Israel TV network has claimed.[31] ABC News had earlier covered the story on 9th of April: that in November a US National Centre for Medical Intelligence report had warned that there was an 'out of control disease' in Wuhan whose 'consequences could be catastrophic.' A Pentagon spokesman denied that any such report had existed.

That was more than a month before the clusters of infection in China started to be reported! The Chinese became aware of the problem around mid- to late December. To quote Kevin Barrett here, "If US intelligence knew that there was a potentially catastrophic pandemic developing in Wuhan, China, in November, it means US intelligence knows what's happening in Wuhan, China, better than the Chinese do. And the only reason that that would be the case would be if the US had planted the virus there." Its reason for doing that he explained was that "the US desperately needs to stop the rise of China to number one world power status."[32]

Also in November - synchronously enough – CEPI, co-founded by Bill Gates a couple of years earlier, pledged $700 million to develop new vaccine platforms, especially for 'disease X' an unknown pathogen. It looked forward to developing a new type of vaccine that tampered with human DNA, this being the precise month in which C19 infection was actually germinating in Wuhan - although the world did not yet know that. The *Coalition for Epidemic Preparedness Innovations* was developing a huge momentum with far-reaching global connections. A year earlier it had developed its fateful collaboration with Imperial College to achieve its goal. To quote Vanessa Beeley, 'One year before the Covid-19 outbreak, Imperial College was working on a vaccine for 'Disease X.'[33] This

---

[31] Israel's i24 news website; Press TV 18 April'US notified Israel about coronavirus in mid-November: Israeli TV'
[32] K.B., Veterans Today, 20 April 'Did US torpedo the entire global economy to stop China's rise?'
[33] Ukcolumn.org Vanessa Beeley 6 May, 'The Big Pharma players behind UK Government lockdown.'

new vaccine-developing platform was called 'RapidVac.' The very department that frightened the British people into a lockdown, had received grant money for developing a vaccine to counter it. On January 17th of 2020, the various groups that had been rehearsing for the pandemic issued their 'Joint call to action' to world governments.[34] Issued jointly by the The John Hopkins Center for Health Security, the World Economic Forum and the Gates foundation, it opened with the categorical claim that disaster was about to strike: 'The next severe pandemic will not only cause great illness and loss of life but could also trigger major cascading

Imperial College London

Home | College and Campus | Science | Engineering | Health | Bus

Tailor-made flu and Disease X vaccines to be created in $8 million project

by Kate Wighton
10 December 2018

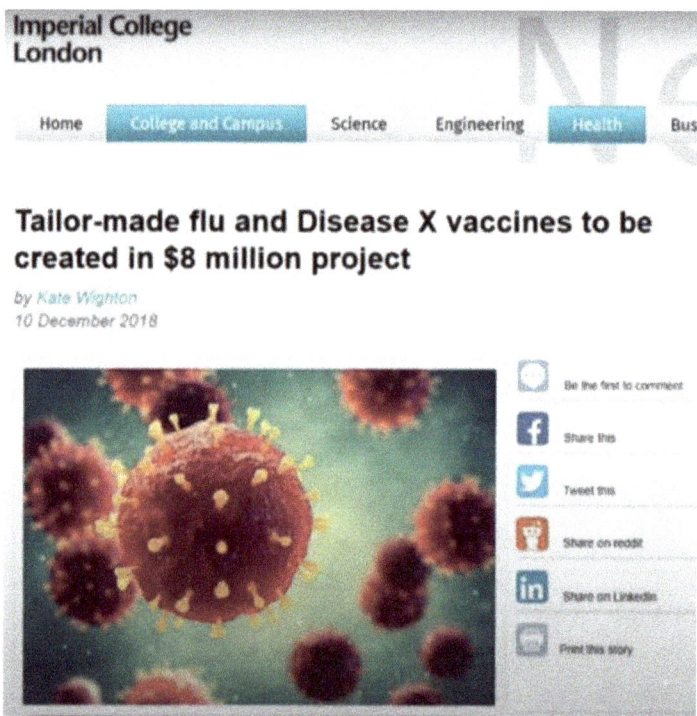

economic and societal consequences that could contribute greatly to global impact and suffering.' This, the final version of their various

[34] https://www.centerforhealthsecurity.org/ Center News 17 Jan.

Figure: Imperial college department receives Bill gates' donation in 2018. Note the all-purpose virus image.

recommendations, was put merely days before lockdown in Wuhan. Thus we see a seamless join between the imagining of and preparation for the event in America, and the 'real thing' taking place.

One week before the UK government made its decision, the Imperial College paper was published, endorsing everything in the 'Event 201' agenda. The US or globalist agenda suddenly arrived in the UK with that paper, ostensibly co-written by 31 authors. How could any politician resist its call to action? If we look back at an earlier announcement of its work in Neil Ferguson's department, (see figure) we can see how at the end of 2018 it received a huge grant - and it was from 'CEPI' funded by Bill Gates - to promote vaccine work. It would develop vaccines for a new brand of flu ('Tailor-made flu') and the image looks suspiciously like coronavirus! The virus textbook cover of 2016 here shown is an all-purpose fantasy virus image being used to fool us.

On April 12th Bill Gates appeared on the BBC's flagship *Breakfast* program, and was allowed an unprecedented

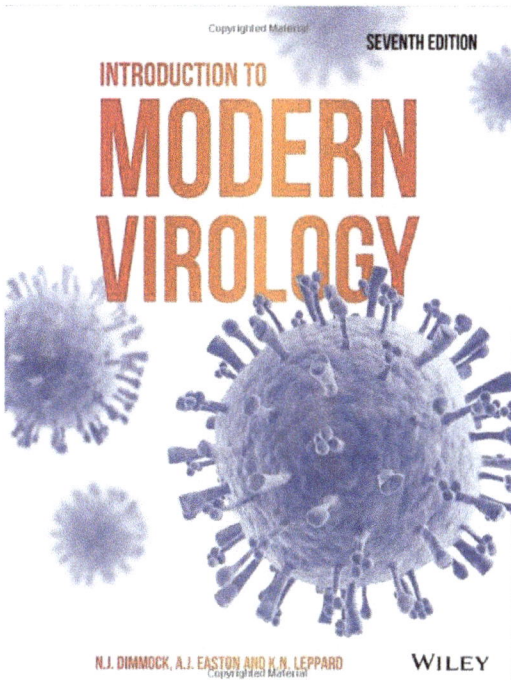

SEVENTH EDITION
INTRODUCTION TO
MODERN
VIROLOGY
N.J. DIMMOCK, A.J. EASTON AND K.N. LEPPARD   WILEY

17

minutes. He was advising the British people that the lockdown should continue until he, Bill Gates, developed the vaccine. He alone could develop it – and this is on the BBC! Gates is here attempting an exact re-run with what he did with Microsoft, whereby much of the world had to end up buying his software and then getting each upgrade. Why did Britain's Chief Medical Officer allow this? Chris Whitty was given the position of the UK's Chief Medical Officer in October 2019, and years earlier in 2008 he had been awarded a £31 million grant from Bill Gates for malaria research.

Bill Gates is developing the ID2020 concept, to give us just what we all need, a 'digital identity.' He is being assisted here by the Rockefeller Foundation and the United Nations. Just a little chip, and it will record if you've been vaccinated or recovered from C19 using 'quantum-dot tattoos'. Bill Gates' website has allowed comments and a remarkable intensity of rage and invective has been piling up in these comment sections! This is, one feels, the voice of the Human Race.

We are reminded of Karl Rove's famous remark (which he later denied of course, but I reckon he said it):

> We're an empire now, and when we act, we create our own reality. And while you're studying that reality – judiciously, as you will – we'll act again, creating other new realities, which you can study too, and that's how things will sort out. We're history's actors . . . and you, all of you, will be left to just study what we do." (Ron Suskind, *NYTimes Magazine*, Oct. 17, 2004).

Has the Empire now 'created its own reality' with a fiendish new bioweapon? If so 'blowback' is the word as it seethes in America! Its hard to see who is benefitting here: computer security software firms and the pharmaceutical industry perhaps. Bill Gates remarked that: 'for the world at large, normalcy only returns when we've largely vaccinated the entire global population.' (*Financial Times* interview,

April 8th) Can you see it coming, vaccine 2.0 followed by vaccine 3.0, etc?

Summarising, it is unequivocally clear that the global event of the year 2020 was conceived and gestated within America and nowhere else. Of interest here is the way the US deaths ie total overall mortality has remained at 5% *below* average compared to previous years – it did not have the big peak after lockdown that happened in the UK. It is a remarkable testimony to the power of American fantasy and American dreaming that the image of a dreadful scourge was sustained. Hospitals were paid for every C19 death registered which helped to sustain the image. One American in six thousand was perceived as having died from C19 – and it was worth shutting down the country for that?

Week	No. Deaths 2019	No. Deaths 2020
1	58,291	59,087
2	58,351	59,151
3	58,194	57,616
4	57,837	57,000
5	58,128	56,426
6	58,492	56,962
7	57,917	55,981
8	57,858	55,494
9	57,920	54,834
10	58,490	54,157
11	57,872	52,198
12	57,087	51,602
13	56,672	52,285
14	56,595	49,292
15	55,477	47,574 => 10 April
TOTAL	865,181	819,659

from: Center for Disease Control

See how the totals actually decrease once the alleged 'pandemic' had been unleashed! Americans, watching their TV screens, would not have been told this.

'Our Coronavirus Catastrophe as Biowarfare Blowback' – that was a brilliant article by Ron Unz published on his unz.com site, America's top intellectual-political discussion site. It may have received more comment and discussion than any other article on that site. In May, a month after it was published, Google de-ranked the entire site – it can no longer be found by searching on Google! Try putting that title into Google and you will not get the unz.com website. If you use the Russian search-engine Yandex it comes up top, as it should do. Deleting videos of the world's most popular speaker, David Icke, is one thing, but removing links to the vast unz.com website is something else, indicating a much darker level of censorship. Unz.com had been enjoying record-breaking traffic until the end of April when Facebook banned it, and it lost some 20% of its traffic, then it was banned on both Google and Facebook. That is to be sure an argument in favour of this little book being produced, where What Really Happened can be remembered and documented.

4

What Happened in Wuhan?

Eyes of Darkness by Dean Koontz (1981) featured a Chinese military lab outside of the city of Wuhan, where a deadly virus was invented as part of the country's biological weapons warfare programme. It was named 'Wuhan-400,' or at least it was given that name in a 1989 reissue of the book: 'Wuhan-400 is a perfect weapon. It afflicts only human beings...' It featured a Chinese scientist who defected to the US, carrying details of this deadly new bio-weapon.

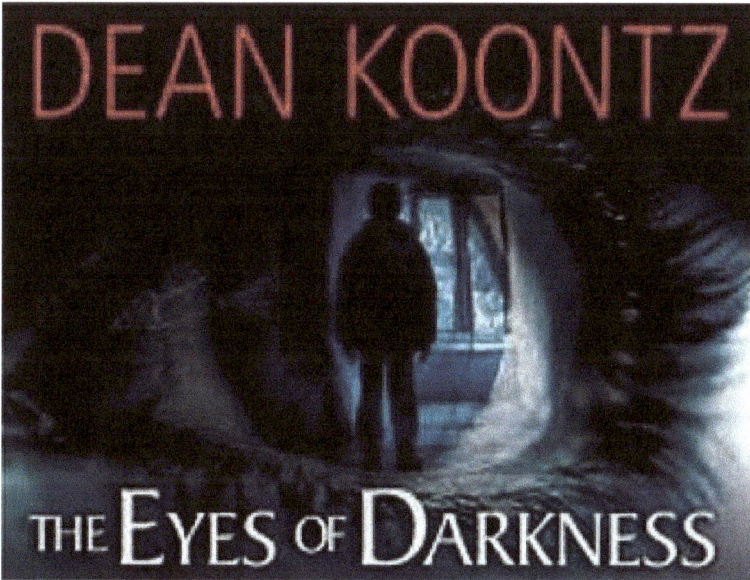

The US Defence Advanced Projects Research Agency DARPA had been funding studies in and near China that discovered new, mutant coronaviruses originating from bats. It spent $10 million on one project in 2018 "to unravel the complex causes of bat-borne viruses that have recently made the jump to humans, causing concern among global health officials." There were a lot of stories about the Pentagon's quest for ethnic-specific bioweapons. Thus,

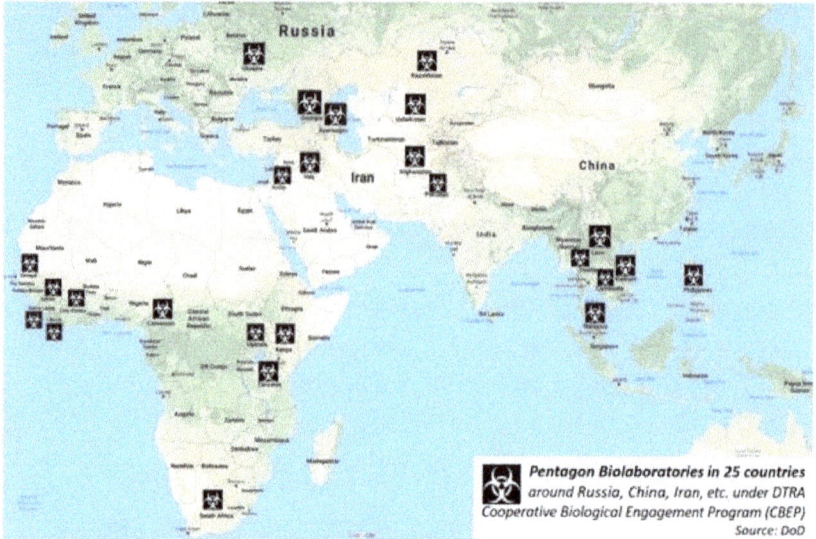

Pentagon Biolaboratories in 25 countries around Russia, China, Iran, etc. under DTRA Cooperative Biological Engagement Program (CBEP)
Source: DoD

"Bio warfare scientists using diplomatic cover test man-made viruses at Pentagon bio laboratories in 25 countries across the world".[35] These US 'scientists' – or we could preferably call them, *necro-technocrats* - have regularly been producing deadly viruses, bacteria and toxins in direct violation of the UN Convention on the Prohibition of Biological Weapons. Also they were developing controversial DNA and mRNA vaccines for a particular coronavirus strain, even though it was a category of vaccine never previously approved for human use in the United States. DARPA had developed ties to the virology institute in Wuhan, China.

[Note: DNA is double-stranded, lives in cell nuclei and can duplicate itself ie reproduce, whereas RNA is usually single-stranded, found in viruses and cannot duplicate itself. mRNA means 'messenger RNA.']

China has been tormented by a series of mystery virus outbreaks. During 2018 and previous years a new 'bird flu' virus swept the country, decimating large portions of China's chicken industry; Chinese scientists claimed that this was a biological warfare event

[35] Sott.net Pentagon Biological-weapon program never ended: US Bio-labs around the world''

but no-one took much notice. Then during 2019 a new Swine Flu viral epidemic devastated China's pig farms, destroying 40% of the nation's primary domestic source of meat - with widespread claims that the latter disease was being spread by mysterious small drones. *Four hundred million pigs* were lost - the largest-ever bio-weapon impact event. That coincided with an escalating US trade war with China and with the western-instigated Hong Kong 'pro-democracy' riots. It peaked in August, exactly when the *Operation Crimson Contagion* drill exercise for the 2020 pandemic was happening in New York.

A 2018 survey of 'trust' showed China had become one of the most trustworthy nations, while the US not surprisingly had sunk down to near the bottom of the list. China was rapidly becoming the Number One economic power in the world and there seemed to be no stopping its wonderful new 'Silk Road' world-trade initiative.

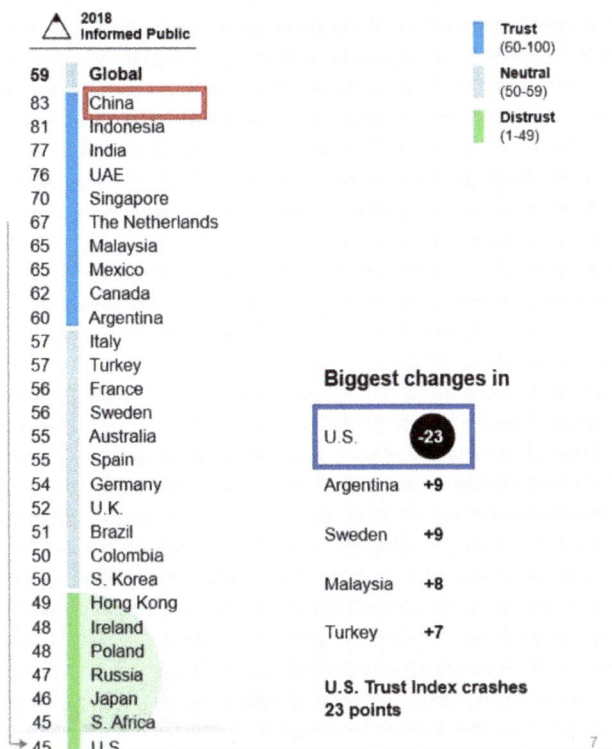

2018 Informed Public

59	Global
83	China
81	Indonesia
77	India
76	UAE
70	Singapore
67	The Netherlands
65	Malaysia
65	Mexico
62	Canada
60	Argentina
57	Italy
57	Turkey
56	France
56	Sweden
55	Australia
55	Spain
54	Germany
52	U.K.
51	Brazil
50	Colombia
50	S. Korea
49	Hong Kong
48	Ireland
48	Poland
47	Russia
46	Japan
45	S. Africa
45	U.S

Trust (60-100)
Neutral (50-59)
Distrust (1-49)

Biggest changes in

U.S. -23
Argentina +9
Sweden +9
Malaysia +8
Turkey +7

U.S. Trust Index crashes 23 points

Clearly, something had to be done! It was developing a reputation for reliability and integrity, and such virtuous behaviour could not go unpunished. On 18th October 2019 the Bill Gates 'Event 201' game-simulation in New York foretold the deadly global *coronavirus epidemic which spread from bats*. That exactly synchronized with the Military World Games held in Wuhan, also on 18th October in which the US team performed so poorly that the Chinese hosts suspected they were not serious! It surmised that they must have had some other purpose, maybe infecting Wuhan with a deadly new bio-weapon virus. This new virus seemed not to target children and people wondered if it was race-specific?

The delegation of 300 U.S. military athletes which arrived in Wuhan in mid-October to participate in the 2019 Military World games stayed in the Wuhan Oriental hotel, right next to the Huanan seafood market (see map). It was around here that the first cluster in Wuhan appeared, of persons diagnosed with C19. Forty-two employees of the Oriental Hotel were diagnosed with C19, that being the first cluster in Wuhan, when only seven people from the seafood market had been diagnosed as C19 positive: all of which had had contact with the 42 from the hotel. (Source:alethonews.com,

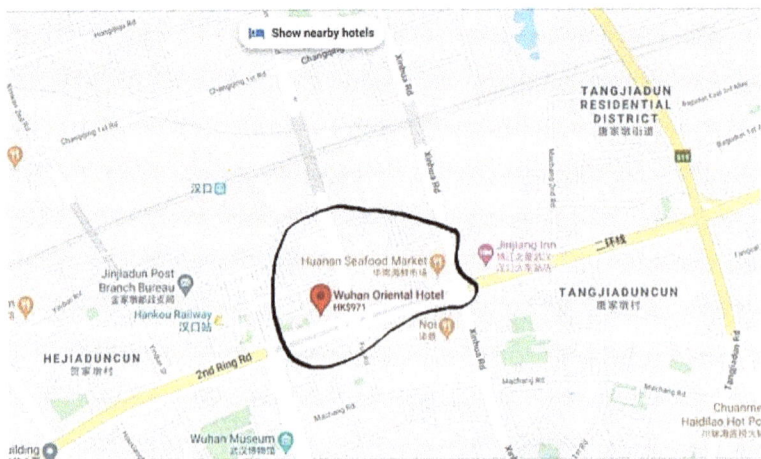

Figure: Map of the seafood market area of Wuhan

22.3.20 'China Demands an Honest Accounting'). From this source, the virus may have spread to the rest of China.

The American Military Games team had trained at a location near Fort Detrick, that being the US military's virology research lab, which was closed down by the Centre of Disease Control in July for various deficiencies. As Ron Unz remarked, "how would Americans react if 300 Chinese military officers had paid an extended visit to Chicago, and soon afterward a mysterious and deadly epidemic had suddenly broken out in that city?"[36] Here's a good comment from an ageing microbiologist:

> It could have been released during the 7th CISM military games held in Wuhan October 18-27, 2019 and that fits perfectly into the time scale for the actual infections. Rumor is that the US participants at CISM were atrocious which is very atypical so one wonders who these "athletes" were. I am reminded of the US military mission in Brazil to help flood victims which coincidentally was the exact same time that all the power transmission stations in Venezuela were destroyed.[37]

The American team did so badly that they were called "Soy Sauce Soldiers" by the Chinese. Many never attended any events and remained close to the Huanan wholesale seafood market. After the American military team returned home on October 28, then within two weeks (the viral incubation period) the first cases of human contact with COVID 19 were ascertained in Wuhan. Many athletes fell ill with a powerful and anomalous influence from which they could not easily recover. The French pentathlete Elodie Clouvel told just such a story to the television station *Loire7* and the Italian swordsman Matteo Tagliariol (Treviso fencing champion and Olympic gold champion in Beijing 2008) confirmed it to local

---

[36] Unz.com, 'American Pravda: Our Coronavirus Catastrophe as Biowarfare Blowback?' 21 April
[37] Thesaker.is 'Old Microbiologist' 12.3.20

newspapers. There were rumours from Intel sources about nano-drones being used thanks to CIA infiltrators: DragonflEye, the light-guided cyber-dragonfly for reconnaissance flights and Black Hornet 3 a micro-helicopter in use by the US army.[38]

The world got to hear about the Chinese city of Wuhan, as the new message of fear emerged in January. Those Chinese had 'wet markets' and the (untrue) story was put out, that they sold live bats to eat. *Something* hit Wuhan rather suddenly but that's about all people can agree on. China has accused the USA of importing it as a bio-weapon while the US President keeps blaming China for it.

Wuhan has a reputation for thick air pollution, and by clearing the sky its lockdown probably saved thousands of lives. More importantly, Wuhan was *the* primary test-city for Chinese installation of 5G everywhere with about ten thousand masts all around the city, and it was fully switched on by November 1st, synchronizing with the outbreak (Chapter 6).

Dr. Francis Boyle had drafted the Biological Weapons Act and was professor of international law at the University of Illinois' law college. He stated that the 2019 Wuhan 'Coronavirus-19' is an *offensive bio-warfare weapon,* and surmised that the infectious disease may have escaped from the Biosafety Level 4 laboratory (BSL-4) outside Wuhan. That Institute of Virology outside Wuhan is the only declared site in China capable of working with deadly viruses. He rejected the idea that it had escaped from the seafood market as the media were alleging. Chinese research scientists claim to have analyzed 27 genomes of the C19 virus and thereby determined that the "most recent common ancestor" for the coronavirus could be dated back to October 1, 2019. Thus we're told, 'Chinese medical authorities and intelligence agencies conducted a rapid and wide-ranging search for the origin of the virus, collecting nearly 100

---

[38] See the site gospanews.net, articles by Fabio Giuseppe Carlo Carisio on CoronaVirus BioWeapon.

samples of the genome from 12 different countries on four continents, identifying all the varieties and mutations. During this research, they determined the virus outbreak had begun much earlier, probably in November, shortly after the Wuhan Military Games. They then came to the same independent conclusions as the Japanese researchers – that the virus did not begin in China but was introduced there from the outside.' [39]

Here is the view of a US ex-bioweapon worker with some experience in this area:

> **Eric Feigl-Ding** ✓
> @DrEricDing
>
> Replying to @DrEricDing
>
> 9. BOTTOMLINE: 1) Seafood market not the source. 2) This RNA #coronavirus mutates really fast. 3) 🦠 has unusual middle segment never seen before in any coronavirus. 4) Not from recent mixing. 5) That mystery middle segment encodes protein responsible for entry into host cells.
>
> ♡ 3,048   5:15 AM - Jan 28, 2020   ⓘ

I have no reason to doubt the Chinese on this, that it originated outside of China and it seems likely to have originated in the US. If, in fact, the US has 5 strains currently and China only one then it must have been percolating in the US for some time before it arose in China…engineered strains are generally unstable over multiple passages through multiple hosts. The worst strains are always those recovered from humans who died from the disease and not field collected strains... If this was perceived to be a useful agent by the likes of Bolton or Pompeo, who are terrible and evil people, then it is

[39] Scott Ritter, 'The Staggering Collapse of US Intelligence on the CoronaVirus' *The American Conservative* 24.3.20. See Corbett Report, 'Was there Foreknowledge of the Pandmic?' 13.4.20

conceivable this was thought to teach the Chinese a lesson in economics. You have to be a complete idiot to release a virus for which you have no effective countermeasures but this administration seems to be filled with complete idiots.

I will also like to add that not all biological warfare agents are lethal. In fact, the worst are non-lethal as it consumes vast amounts of resources in treatment and lost productivity. Deaths are actually cheaper. So, a high communicability, low lethality disease is perfect for ruining an economy.

I believe there were at least two attacks with Iran being the second and perhaps North Korea as well.[40]

Absurd billion-dollar lawsuits are being drummed up by various states of America to sue China on the grounds that it started this modern plague and failed to inform the world of what was happening. Germany too has joined in, as if China could be sued. Here we need to review the time-sequence through which the 'pandemic' has developed.

There was both an ABC news report and also an Israeli Intel report revealing that 'as far back as late November' of 2019 the National Centre for Medical Intelligence was warning of a new virulent contagion in Wuhan getting out of hand.[41] This information had allegedly been gained from wire and computer intercepts plus satellite images. If indeed that warning of a 'potentially catastrophic' pandemic had been given, it was one month too early.

A more recent account has US Intel warning that what was happening in November in Wuhan 'could be a cataclysmic event' as regards the infection, which sounds somewhat exaggerated.[42] At any rate this is tending to endorse what has been claimed by the Chinese

[40] Thesaker.is 'Old Microbiologist' 12.3.20
[41] See 'COVID Was a US Biowar Attack on China, US Intel Knew About It 2 Months Before China Did,' Pepe Escobar, 23.4.20, truthtopowernews.com

[42] Russia Today, What did they know, exactly? US intel warned of 'cataclysmic' coronavirus pandemic in NOVEMBER 2019, report claims 8 April

foreign policy spokesman Lijian Zhao, that it was the Americans who brought the infection to the Wuhan games.

China identified the new disease on December 30th, that being when their first Sars-Covid-19 case was detected. This information was duly communicated to the WHO and then on January 3rd the head of the American Centre for Disease Control Robert Redfield called the top Chinese CDC official to discuss the matter. Then Chinese doctors set about sequencing the virus. A couple of months later, Chinese scientists managed to positively trace back their first real case of Sars-Covid-19 to November 17th.

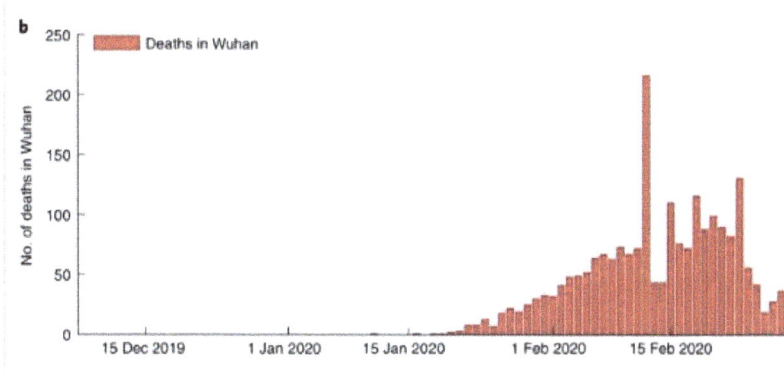

How did America have that foreknowledge? The finger of accusation points at this being a US 'op.' Thus the US Secretary of State Mike Pompeo has described it as a 'live exercise:' "This is not about retribution," Pompeo explained at a mid-March White House briefing, "This matter is going forward — we are in a live exercise here to get this right"; to which an annoyed-looking President can be heard replying, 'You should have let us know.' He was muttering under his breath however the recording has been amplified and those are his words. That was on March 20th.

Thus the US is trying to imply that the Wuhan lab created the C19 bioweapon and so is responsible for it coming to the USA. America is a country that always needs a foreign enemy, whereby it is able to project onto the Other that which it is itself doing, and so the Other can be blamed, hated and demonised with impunity.

Whatever China 'got' or caught was absurdly small, compared to the western nations -

Nation	Total CV deaths	Pop^n	Deaths/m
UK	34,636	56.1m	617
US	91,730	331m	277
China	4634	1.41 bn	3

(for May 17th, 2000)

On April 6th Wuhan re-opened its industries, even as the CV-19 incidence in the UK and US kept climbing.

5

Of Viruses and Exosomes

What is a virus? Nowadays we may hope that a message will 'go viral' and by that we mean travel and self-multiply, spreading itself via different 'hosts.' Also, there are the 'viruses' that get into computers and insert rogue instructions, so that the programs no longer work properly. These modern usages greatly colour our perception.

But are they really like that, do they have such permanence and can they travel across the world? We all think we've seen pictures of the C19 virus, however viruses are *not* seen down an electron microscope. The 'PCA' test for C19 is able to identify a virus-like sequence of bases on a DNA strand, where 'bases' are the units of the genetic code. Or, a test for antibodies will detect certain proteins, and it is inferred from them that there must be some invading virus.[43] But are these inferences sound?

The epidemiologist Dr Andrew Kaufman and author Janine Roberts have suggested a different approach, which may help to separate out faulty assumptions.[44] We quote here from Roberts' book *Fear of the Invisible,* and you might feel this is the first time these things have ever made sense.

> Cells make particles that travel though 'extra cellular space' to other cells, not to 'perniciously infect' them but to pass information onto them. Cells 'talk ' to one another. The genome is modified by absorbing in part codes created by other cells.

This is a process of communication.

---

[43] https://www.newmedicineonline.com/viruses/
[44] Janine Roberts, *Fear of the Invisible How scared should we be of Viruses and Vaccines,* 2008

Today, many biologists are no longer automatically naming all such travelling elements as 'viruses.' Many of them are now called vesicles' a name widely used since 1997. These are generically described as 'cargo loaded small vesicles released into extra-cellular space.'

They carry information, in the form of RNA:

As viruses do not usually survive longer than a few days and cannot reproduce themselves, cells must be constantly making and sending out an enormous number of them.. Cells, whether healthy or sick, are constantly making vesicles or viruses, but virology textooks normally start their description of virus production from when a virus is about to infect a cell. .. If it is universally accepted that cells make every virus that exists, so why not start from where this process starts, from when a living cell creates messenger RNA with instructions to encode and make a virus?

'Exosomes' are produced by cells and excreted by them:

All kinds of cells make exosomes…When near tumour cells, exosomes are reported to sometimes produce very strong anti-tumour reactions. Radiation-damaged cells also produce exosomes, perhaps as a genetic code repair mechanism.

Exosomes are now called 'one of the most important protein complexes' involved in controlling the 'RNA-processing machinery' in mammals. They vitally help ensure accuracy in the reading of RNA messages and help deactivate old RNA messages that are no longer needed. Like the virus they contain RNA:

In 2007 it was described how cells 'send RNA messages to each other by packing these into exosomes' and how exosomes can carry a a 'large amount of DNA' from one cell to another.

This RNA can sometimes be double-stranded, like DNA:

In the first stage the cell encodes information in the form of a strand or double strand of DNA or RNA. It then surrounds this with a protective capsid of protein, plus sometimes a membrane envelope as well, before sending it out from the cell. On arrival at another cell, its genetic strands and proteins are brought inside that cell and absorbed. After this, the virus no longer exists. Any new virus or vesicle is made afresh.

They are de-activated when no longer required:

When viruses arrive at the cell, the code they contribute is immediately assessed, and may then be silenced by mRNAs in a process known as 'RNA interference.'

How does this work in epidemics or disease? She doubts the conventional theory:

Viruses have no metabolism so they cannot produce energy or eat.. they have no nervous system, no sensory system, no intelligence that can facilitate any kind of invasion or the hijacking of a cell a billion times larger. The conventional theory of viral hijacking is that, after the short genetic code of a virus has been absorbed by a cell, the 'viral genes' absorbed start to 'direct the production of proteins by the host cellular machinery.' It is assumed they are able to force the host cell to do this… But I had to ask, would cells give such minute and 'dead' messenger vesicles the extraordinary ability to pirate cells of the same organism?.. if cells create viruses as weapons against other cells.. then this would be remarkably suicidal as viruses usually pass from cell to cell within the same organism.

The whole theory seemed unlikely to her:

Many virologists have been driven to speak of viruses as if they possess the cleverness of the cell (and thus as if they were bacteria.).. modern virology is built upon the idea that viruses invade and destroy… the virus absorbed on arrival at a cell is nothing much more than food and information for the cell… most epidemics were ended by the provision of good hygiene, pure water and adequate food before these vaccines were invented… Are similar viruses found in similar diseases because cells respond with a very similar message in response to the same challenge?

If cells get sick, damaged or malnourished, that will tend to be *before* the viruses are detected. The viruses aren't *causing* anything:

…It thus seems that cells may be sick, poisoned, stressed or malnourished in some way before they show the symptoms of 'viral infection.' There is a considerable body of evidence that indicates cellular illness or malnourishment often precedes the production of viruses, rather than the converse…. I have found to my surprise that scientists have long known that the guaranteed way to make cells produce viruses in the laboratory, including flu and measles virus, is not primarily by getting them infected, but by exposing them to stress and toxins!

Do viruses spread disease? We're told that flu can be spread by people coughing, however she found a textbook about how experiments had been unable to show this:

transmission experiments from people infected with a rhinovus to susceptibles sitting opposite at a table proved singularly unsuccessful. Equally unsuccessful was the transmission of influenza from a naturally infected husband/wife to his/her spouse.[45]

Thus concerning the common cold virus,

The symptoms of a cold are associated with at least 200 different types of virus … All that can be said for certain is that during colds we produce a multitude of different viruses.

---

[45] *Introduction to Modern Virology* by N.Dimmock & S. Primrose, 2016, Blackwell Science, p.230.

Next time you 'catch' a cold, try not to assume that it's because of a 'virus' that has somehow got into you. While your body is trying to recover, tiny inter-cellular messages will be flowing about that can be called 'viruses.'

> ..what Dr Steven Lanks a virologist had controversially reported ..he could find no evidence for the complete isolation of any pathogenic virus. He then went one step further. He interpreted the electron micrographs published of 'viruses' as solely showing parts of the 'intra- and intercellular transport' system -such as the vesicles. He said viruses were thus 'cell components.'

We need, she concludes, to abandon the modern 'enemy' theory as if we always have to be at war with something:

> The mythology surrounding viruses is deeply misleading. They are frequently targeted and described as intelligent enemies that deserve to have a multi-billion dollar 'war on terror' waged against them- to the great benefit of the pharmaceutical industry... Surely it is time to leave behind this ugly obsession with unseen dangers – particularly from what are nothing more or less than cellular messengers.'

The words of her final paragraph are especially relevant:

> And don't let anyone use fear to manipulate you.

That perspective helps us to appraise the view of the naturopathic doctor Andrew Kaufman. His video 'Is COVID-19 really an Exosome not a virus?' [46] has been endorsed by quite a few of the most intelligent critiques of the whole C19 story. His Youtube statement is here paraphrased.

Within cells, what are called exosomes transfer genetic material in the form of messenger RNAs to make proteins and micro-RNAs. These regulate the expression of genes. Exosomes are small

---

[46] Kaufman 'What I think COVID-19 really is' 16 April

membrane vesicles secreted by most cell types. The coronavirus story has been misunderstood, starting from when Chinese scientists took liquid from people's lungs and found 'genetic material' including some RNA.

There will always be free genetic material circulating around blood and body fluids and all sorts of things will contain such, eg normal bacteria. The scientists determined its 'sequence' ie the code of the genetic material and then they rushed to develop a diagnostic test (a PCR, 'polymerase chain reaction'). This tests for a sequence of RNA, which may be present in a virus but also in various other things.

As Kary Mullis inventor of the PCR test explained, 'these tests cannot detect free, infectious viruses at all…The tests can detect genetic sequences of viruses, but not viruses themselves.'[47]

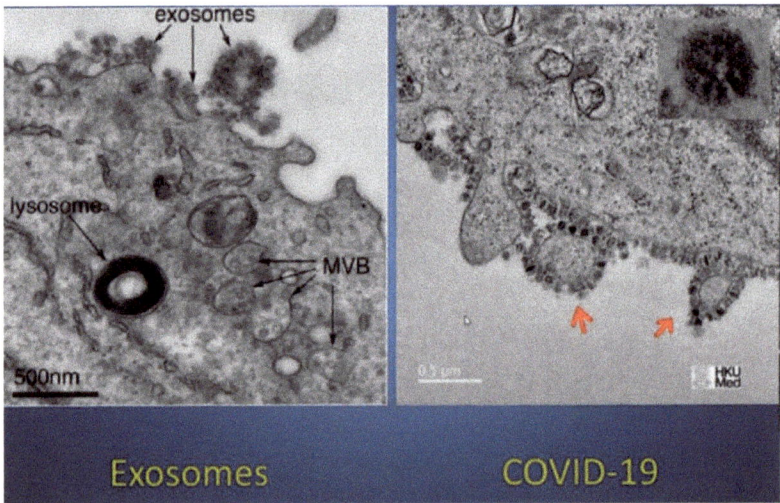

Figure: Dr Kaufman compares what is alleged to be a C19 image with exosomes, using electron microscope images (20,000x magnification).

---

[47] www.virusmyth.com/aids/hiv/jlprotease.htm 9.12.96

They wrongly applied this test *before* they had purified the virus. The supposed 'COVID-19' virus has never been purified and visualised. What is called a 'gold standard' i.e. the purified substance was never found or ascertained. In theory the PCR test should be compared with such a 'gold standard' and also a control group that has no such virus - that essential test was never done. The PCR test goes through cycles of doubling the RNA, maybe 25-30 times, until there is enough to measure. A slight mistake will generate false positives and the test produces many of these.

Exosomes are naturally-occurring in the body and may bud out from a cell. Here is an electron microscope picture (with kind permission) where Kaufman compared them to the alleged coronavirus.

They are he claims *the exact same thing*. He found a quote by a distinguished medical virology expert James Hildreth who wrote in relation to HIV studies, 'The virus is fully an exosome in every sense of the word.' Exosomes are produced and thrown out of cells by insults to the body, eg toxins, shock and fear, ionizing radiation and so forth. They are the same size, about five hundred nanometres in

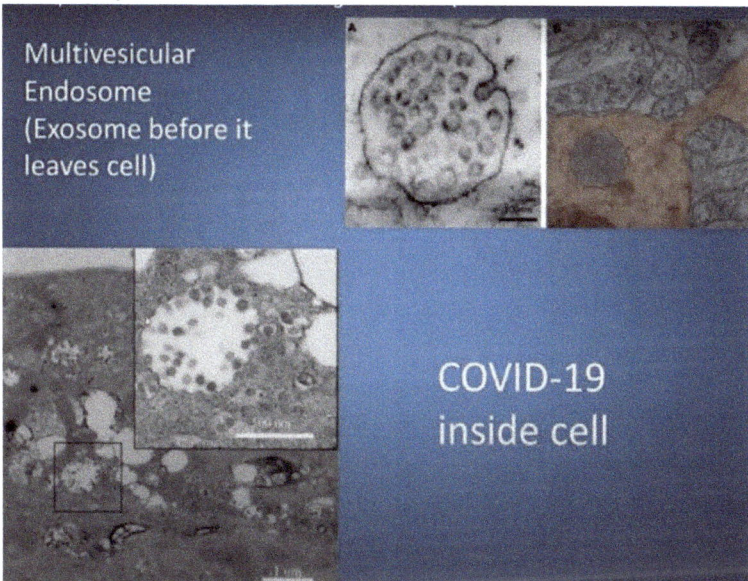

diameter, both have only RNA and no DNA and both are found in lung tissue. Exosomes have the same 'lock and key' process as the receptor part of the virus, whereby it enters the cell.

Here is one more picture he used showing the exosome *inside* a cell. A lot of people seem to be endorsing the Kaufman view, that the pictures we've been shown of 'COVID-19' are actually tiny 'exosome' entities produced within the cell.

Chinese scientists had sampled lung tissue fluid and found that lung cancer cells were making exosomes. Excreted by cells these have the function of swallowing up little toxin particles as a sort of clean-up broom and thereby help the cell to survive. By putting out the exosome the cell promotes its survival. It thus looks as if the exosome is helping to clear away toxins. They are a reaction to the real cause of illness. There are some twenty different illnesses that will produce a cough, fever and lower white blood count, Like a sponge the exosomes will soak up toxins. In summary, *there is no pandemic*: the numbers are far too low. But, there is some sort of affliction going on, and exosomes result from the lung insult/damage.

Detecting the virus

There is, we gather, a simple test to ascertain whether you have been infected. If you have a raised temperature, or if you can't hold your breath for ten seconds without coughing, you are liable to be asked to take a so-called 'PCR' test. But, this test seems to have the characteristic, that however many times it is explained, however much you read about it, it never quite makes sense. It involves getting DNA from your body to replicate and multiply, and this method was invented by the late Kary Mullis in 1983, for which he was awarded the Nobel Prize. But, how one infers therefrom the presence of an alleged C19 virus is never made clear.

We'd assume that someone somewhere would have done the following simple and basic experiment. John Rappaport realised that the following would be proper starting-point – *if* any real science was going on. Take two groups of people, one sick and the other healthy, and let samples be taken from them with swabs, and let the PCR test be run on them blind, so that those doing the test don't know who is ill or healthy. Then when the results come out, how well do these correlate with the sick / healthy individuals? Do they, at all? Surely, they would, we'd assume? Well, don't bet on it. Secondly, if there is perchance some degree of correlation, we'd expect several different labs to do the tests, to see how well – or if at all - the different laboratory results agree?

But surely, you will say, that must have been done? That's basic science. John Rappaport concluded: 'In the absence of this experiment, the quantitative PCR must be looked at as a rogue hypothesis that should never have been foisted on the public in the first place.'[48]

We're endlessly shown pictures of the alleged virus. You could be forgiven for supposing, that samples were taken from a number of people who seem to have the mystery new illness, and these were purified and then scrutinised under an electron microscope; and that *similar* tiny 'viruses' were seen in such samples; whereas these tended not to be present in samples from healthy persons. Again this *has not been done.*

As Mr Rappaport so rightly observes, 'It's essential to realize where the burden of proof rests.' Those telling us that some new disease or new virus exits, surely ought to have done these extremely simple and rudimentary experiments.

---

[48] Rappaport, COVID: 'Two basic experiments that have never been done' 29 April nomorefakenews.com. For further insight see interview with Dr Andrew Kaufman: 'They Want to Genetically Modify us with C19' Vaccine' 10th May.

Citizens all around the world *believe* in the lockdown, in social distancing and in wearing facemasks. Normally, no-one can get an entire population to agree upon something, let alone the whole world. Could some evidence be relevant here? If one could show for example that people wearing a facemask when going outdoors were less likely to get ill than those who did not, then that would show something: and you may be sure we would have heard it by now - together with nonstop ethical censure of 'those irresponsible people' who did not wear them. But, we haven't. Likewise, if persons who had been enjoying walks in the park etc instead of properly self-isolating were tending more to test positive for C19, then surely we'd have heard it by now – but we haven't. Rather the contrary in fact - see last chapter. This rudimentary, basic science *just is not there.*

Don't wear a facemask

Advice against wearing facemasks has been given by the US neurosurgeon and health practitioner Dr Russell Blaylock.[49] The WHO has recommended use of a 'N95' face mask to breathe through and the UK government is endorsing this advice. But, no studies have been done to demonstrate that either a cloth mask or the N95 mask has any effect on transmission of the COVID-19 virus. Dr Blaylock advises that 'By wearing a mask, the exhaled viruses will not be able to escape and will concentrate in the nasal passages, enter the olfactory nerves and travel into the brain.' 'While most agree that the N95 mask can cause significant hypoxia and hypercapnia, (raised carbon dioxide in the blood) another study of surgical masks found significant reductions in blood oxygen as well. In this study, researchers examined the blood oxygen levels in 53 surgeons using an oximeter. They measured blood oxygenation before surgery as well as at the end of surgeries'. Thus, researchers found that the mask *reduced* the blood oxygen levels. Dr Blaylock adds,

---

[49] https://jamesfetzer.org/ Dr Blaylock 'Face Masks Pose Serious Risks To The Healthy' 16 May

As for the scientific support for the use of face mask, a recent careful examination of the literature, in which 17 of the best studies were analyzed, concluded that, "None of the studies established a conclusive relationship between mask/respirator use and protection against influenza infection."[50] Keep in mind, no studies have been done to demonstrate that either a cloth mask or the N95 mask has any effect on transmission of the COVID-19 virus. Any recommendations, therefore, have to be based on studies of influenza virus transmission. And, as you have seen, there is no conclusive evidence of their efficiency in controlling flu virus transmission.

There is another danger to wearing these masks on a daily basis, especially if worn for several hours. When a person is infected with a respiratory virus, they will expel some of the virus with each breath. If they are wearing a mask, especially an N95 mask or other tightly fitting mask, they will be constantly rebreathing the viruses, raising the concentration of the virus in the lungs and the nasal passages.

People wear facemasks because they trust the advice which their government gives them . Ah, if only that trust were warranted! There is insufficient evidence that wearing a mask of any kind can have a significant impact in preventing the spread of this virus.

Bill Gates will surely be remembered by his words spoken in mid-April, 'Normalcy only returns when we've largely vaccinated the entire global population.' That is a remarkable declaration about a vaccine that *does not yet exist*: it is *presumed* that it will develop. Such mandatory vaccination will make hundreds of billions of dollars for the likes of Bill Gates.

---

[50] bin-Reza F. et al. 'The use of mask and respirators to prevent transmission of influenza: A systematic review of the scientific evidence'. *Resp Viruses* 2012;6(4):257-67

When it comes to such a vaccine that may soon be mandatory, let us remember the wise words of virology expert Dr Judy Mikovitz *'There is no vaccine currently on the schedule for any RNA virus that works.'* As regards where it originated, she gave what is likely to be the best answer we're going to get: 'I'm sure it originated between the North Carolina laboratories, Fort Dietrich, the US Army Institute of Infectious diseases and the Wuhan Laboratory.' These are quotes from her massively censored interview in the Documentary 'Plandemic.' This 26-minute discussion of real science and fake virology has repeatedly been deleted from Youtube and banned from all internet uploading platforms as well as being denounced and scoffed at by Wikipedia, the *New York Times* and sundry other MSM. In consequence it soon notched up millions of views and, currently up on Bitchute, is probably the most-watched video in Bitchute history! If there's one must-watch video on the topic this is it. That censorship also sent her book rocketing up into the Amazon top ten, briefly gaining the number one position! Plus it made third place in the *New York Times* bestseller list: *Plague of Corruption: Restoring Faith in the Promise of Science.*

That is certainly a topical title, and the reason for the popularity of her video is easy to explain: Dr Mikovitz does know what she's talking about.

****

6

Surrounded by 5G

The synchrony was exact.

On March 12 2020 we were told that in the UK a further twenty-one cities had 'gone live' with 5G, making a total of seventy cities then 'switched on'.

That date can therefore be accepted as the official date for when '5G cities' began to function in the UK.

We then see the following extremely significant dates lying very closely together:

12 March - 5G is switched on in the UK

17 March - Ferguson publishes his computer prediction of half a million UK deaths if the new 'pandemic' is allowed to run its course

23 March – the UK Prime Minister instructs all UK citizens to stay at home.

If we reject the idea that these pivotal steps taking place in such quick succession is pure coincidence, we must then open our minds to the possibility of a hidden hand at work here, with its own agenda, known only to a few.

Looking at the earlier switching on of 5G in Wuhan, China, at the start of October 2019, we can see that the new symptoms we were told were caused by a 'new flu' virus started to appear only a matter of weeks later.

The few, blurry video sequences that were aired, illustrating the symptoms of this new virus in Wuhan, showed people suffering a sudden spasm, shuddering as if they could no longer breathe and then falling to the ground.

The question therefore needs to be posed as to what could have this seemingly instantaneous effect upon the lungs?

In the month of April two things happened, both unprecedented in human history: the lockdown, together with swarms of yellow-clad BT engineers out and about putting up 5G wires and 5G towers. This chapter examines the second of these, which was a covert operation in the sense of being unannounced in the media. An intense Youtube censorship was at once present of any videos suggesting that 5G may be harmful to health, while newspapers scoffed at the deranged 'conspiracy theorists' who were suggesting such a thing. A simple video of, for example, how dead birds have fallen out of a tree, once a 5G antenna was put up next to it – that would tend not to remain up for long.

A Longer View

It is appropriate to step back a bit and gain a perspective of how the development of electricity and especially radio waves have developed, as the 2G, 3G and 4G unfolded with no-one giving a thought as to the biological effect. A rather powerful and I suspect definitive book *The Invisible Rainbow a History of Electricity and Life* has now appeared by Arthur Firstenberg which surveys the whole development over a couple of centuries, and especially the price in terms of health that *homo sap.* is paying. This is a deep, *ecological* treatise about how lifeforms on Planet Earth are interlinked, and the central role played therein by electricity and magnetism, and the sensitivity of all life to different electrical frequencies.

The development of the 'flu' especially concerns us and here are some quotes to give a flavor of this radical new discovery:

"Anxiety disorder," afflicting one-sixth of humanity, did not exist before the 1860s, when telegraph wires first encircled the earth. No hint of it appears in the medical literature before 1866.

Influenza, in its present form, was invented in 1889, along with alternating current. It is with us always, like a familiar guest – so familiar that we have forgotten that it wasn't always so. (p.65)

As living beings, not only do we possess a mind and a body, but we also have nerves that join the two.…..As a network of fine transmission wires, it can readily be damaged or unbalanced by a great or unfamiliar electric load. This has effects on both mind and body that we know today as anxiety disorder.

If influenza is primarily an electrical disease, a response to an electrical disturbance of the atmosphere, then it is not contagious in the ordinary sense. The patterns of its epidemics should prove this, and they do. (p.85)

The embarrassing secret among virologists is that from 1933 until the present day, there have been no experimental studies proving that influenza – either the virus or the disease – is ever transmitted from person to person by normal contact. As we will see in the next chapter, all efforts to experimentally transmit it from person to person, even in the midst of the most deadly disease epidemic the world has ever known, have failed.

From 1933 to the present day, virologists have been unable to present any experimental study proving that influenza spreads through normal contact between people. All attempts to do so have met with failure.

Experiments have *not* succeeded in obtaining a presumed flu virus, giving it to a healthy person, and have them succumb to the illness. Flu-type illnesses do not seem to be transmissable in that manner. We so much take this for granted today that it's hard to imagine otherwise.

Experiments have greatly failed to confirm that diseases can be transmitted by viral infection. Going back a hundred years (to summarise) we saw how, during the deadly 1918/19 flu epidemic, the US Public Health Service collaborated with the Navy using a hundred volunteers who had not previously had the flu. They were first inoculated with what was presumed to be the flu bug, by spraying it into their noses and throats but none of them got ill. Next they did the same with swabs taken from people in hospital with the flu and again no-one got ill. Finally the volunteers were taken into the hospitals and told to mix with flu patients and shake hands with them etc. (Rosenau 1921) and still they didn't get ill. That could be the only genuine investigation into the transmissability or contagion of flu, and it found that a healthy person could not be made to become infected by any kind of contact with an infected person.[51]

In the 20th century, Firstenberg distinguishes three main steps in radio-communication and the flu epidemics that accompanied them.

* In 1918 as the radio era began, it was ushered in by the Spanish influenza pandemic just as WW1 was ending.

* In 1957 as the radar era began it was ushered in by the Asian flu pandemic of that year.

* In 1968 the satellite era began, interfering with the magnetosphere, and that was ushered in by the Hong Kong flu pandemic of 1968.

Doctors noticed that these epidemics would travel too fast for a virus, appearing simultaneously in different places, and then once the flu was over the virus would somehow just … disappear.

In this 21st century, we have grown familiar with electric masts towering over our cities. Firstenberg quotes survey after survey showing how greatly the incidence of cancer varies with the distance of residents from such towers and that victims living closer develop the cancer years earlier. For example, in San Francisco, childhood cancer rate was studied as a function of distance from the Sutro

---

[51] Firstenberg, *The Invisible Rainbow*, p.107-9 (a summary).

Tower. Almost one thousand feet tall, that tower was broadcasting around one million watts of VHF and FM radio signals, plus over 18 million watts of UHF-TV. Children who lived less than one kilometre from the tower had nine times the rate of leukemia, 31 times the rate of brain cancer and 18 times the total cancer rate, compared to children in the rest of the city. That survey was conducted in the year 2000. (p.260)

Brain tumours result from cellphone use but these have been greatly covered up by the industry. Firstenberg describes how difficult it was and still is to get a hold of the data, but nonetheless a Swedish study was able to conclude that 'using both cell phones and cordless phones significantly increases one's risk of brain cancer… the more years you use such a phone and the more cumulative hours you use one and the younger you are at first exposure, the greater the odds that you will develop a tumour.' (p.259) Malignant brain tumours have nowadays become the most common cancer among children aged 10-18, which has never happened before. Attention Deficit Disorder or ADHD increases amongst children in proportion to cell phone use as likewise does hearing loss.

Tinnitus or ringing in the ears is a modern and very much a 21st – century affliction. A Swedish professor of audiology Holgers found in 1997 during routine testing of children that only twelve percent of them had ringing in their ears, whereas more recently in 2004 she found that amongst a group of schoolchildren aged 9 to 16 almost half of them had spontaneous tinnitis. Other studies confirm a worldwide, dramatic increase in tinnitus in populations during the transition into this 21st century (p.320), whereas the phenomenon used to be fairly rare. Firstenburg describes the electric-magnetic nature of the sensors in the ear, in relation to the little hairs of the cochlea, and how high frequencies affect them.

A major cause of this phenomenon could be the 'smart metres' installed into homes:

The wireless version of smart metres .. has spread round the world like technological wildfire in the past few years, rapidly becoming the single most intrusive source of electronic noise in modern life....The meters in a mesh network communicate not only with the utility company but with each other, each meter chattering loudly to its neighbours as frequently as two hundred and forty thousand times a day.' (p318)

Simple Experiments

There is need for a more feminist science which is aware of the Web of Life and how to preserve and not destroy it. If we don't manage that, then future progress is going to be a slow-motion suicide. Thus, concerning EMF safety thresholds there is a vast difference between what might be safe for the developing nervous system of the growing child and for the embryo in the womb, and on the other hand the safety threshold used by industry to define how adults can be exposed during working hours without suffering permanent damage. The latter is based on heating and so long as the EM radiant energy doesn't actually cook the workers – as microwaves in an oven cook food - its deemed to be OK. There seems to be about *six or seven orders of magnitude* difference between these safety levels.

In the UK, the government agency OFCOM measured the EM radiation in inner-city school playgrounds before 5G was switched on (October 2019) and were happy to report that the ambient levels were a mere 1% of the maximal permitted dose.[52] The government agency called Public Health England makes reassuring noises while 5G is being installed,[53] and it cites a similar high safety level.

Appendix 3 describes the search for more sensible safety levels, such as that recommended by 'Create Healthy Homes' or 'The Bio-

---

[52]www.gov.uk/government/publications/5g-technologies-radio-waves-and-health/5g-technologies-radio-waves-and-health
[53]It cites the International Commission on Non-Ionizing Radiation Protection, ICNIRP

Initiative 2012, A Rationale for Biologically-based Exposure standards for low-intensity EM Radiation.' The latter concludes: "Public safety standards are 1,000 – 10,000 or more times higher than levels now commonly reported in mobile phone base station studies to cause bioeffects" and alas that seems to be a sound judgment.

Simple experiments on plants and creatures need to be developed, to try and bring an awareness of what is going on. Most people just blank out if one quotes ambient levels and they can't tell the difference between say milliwatts and microwatts. One can try the experiment of germinating two lots of mustard and cress, one lot having a mobile phone under it, and see the difference. *One grows, the other doesn't.* For practically any seeds I believe that will work. Every school biology program needs to feature such an experiment. The *Mail* ran a report on how 'What's WiFi doing to us? Experiment finds that shrubs die when placed next to Wireless Routers' (6.5.20). That's a good start! A meter can be purchased that will detect ambient EM power strength and a safe level is *that where the growth of the seedlings will not be inhibited.*[54]

A school biology lab needs to be able to observe beehives in a garden. Putting a mobile phone next to a beehive will cause it to empty. Again this is a very simple experiment and, don't worry, the bees will come back again when it is removed. Millennials will never know what is meant by the phrase 'the murmuring of innumerable bees' as they just see the odd lonely bee buzzing around. What will happen to bee colonies once 5G is up and running is too awful to contemplate. A safe level of EM radiation is one that *would not disturb the activity of a beehive.*

Sparrows used to be very common in the UK, and their decimation has followed the rollout of mobile telephony. At the dawn of this century they made it onto the UK's threatened and endangered species list. Kensington Gardens Park in London

[54] Eg, 'Acoustimeter' https://emfields-solutions.com/shop/acoustimeter/

counted 2,603 sparrows in 1925 and that dropped to *just four* in 2002. Sparrows have associated with human beings for thousands of years and their abundance was alluded to by Jesus! But today, even where there are plenty of seeds and insects around, the sparrows have vanished.

In the 19th century canaries were used by miners as a life-or-death safety aid. Down a mine, if the bird died the air was toxic. Surely the birds have a no less urgent message for us today. An experiment with storks in Spanish cities clearly demonstrated the effect of cellphone antennae upon fertility. Sixty of their rooftop nests were selected, thirty within two hundred metres of an antenna and the other thirty at more than three hundred metres away. The near group were exposed to four times stronger radiation on average and hatched only half the number of baby storks, while the birds very close, within a hundred metres, fought while trying to construct the nest and sometimes couldn't even manage that. (p.325)

Why is this result so important? Try to tell people that plummeting levels of human fertility in the entire industrialised world are being *caused by* electromagnetic radiation and you're liable to get some dismissive grin and a comment like, 'Oh, you're one of those conspiracy theorists are you?' because indeed it is hard to prove. 5G could well be a major extinction event in this 21st century with industrialised nations losing their fertility. Africa being not wired up with 5G will remain fertile. But we're digressing somewhat: such an experiment with storks demonstrates in an accepted scientific format that the bird fertility has a strong negative correlation with the EM intensity.

In Germany, local residents have been startled by birds falling from trees. The mysterious, unidentified disease started in March of 2020 and has afflicted many small songbirds across Germany. By April 21 the number of reported sick and/or dead birds was around 26,000. The victims are being described as "apathetic birds with breathing problems," who no longer eat properly and appear to be "unquenchably thirsty" before they die. Extreme thirst is a widely-reported effect of microwave radiation, plus it is also commonly reported in cases of C19.

The regions experiencing the bird-death outbreaks correspond to areas where Vodafone announced in a press release that it had expanded its cell tower network. Vodafone said it had closed "one of the nastiest radio holes" in Lower Saxony, and there had previously only been 2G service along the Mosel River. Basically - Arthur Firstenburg is arguing - there exists a correlation in Germany between mystery bird deaths and upgraded WiFi services: "It is no coincidence that Germany, this spring, brought 4G-LTE technology for the first time to areas near its borders immediately before small birds began dying in large numbers in precisely those areas."[55]

Science Warning

The scientist Dr. Martin Pall (Professor Emeritus of Biochemistry and Basic Medical Sciences at Washington State University) has stated concisely that

> Putting in tens of millions of 5G antennae without a single biological test of safety has got to be about the stupidest idea anyone has had in the history of the world.

He came out with the following 5G predictions, back in December of 2019.[56] When fully turned on, we will see (1) decreased human reproduction, (2) lowered collective brain function, (3) very early-onset Alzheimer's, (4) increased autism and ADHD, (5) deterioration of the human gene pool, and (6) massive increases in cardiac arrests. He has tracked numerous signs of its biological effects, for example, he has outlined increases in neuropsychiatric effects, cardiac effects, and electromagnetic hypersensitivity. As we

---

[55] cellphonetaskforce.org/wp-content/uploads/2020/05/The-Evidence-Mounts.pdf
[56] Search for: 'Massive predictive effects of 5G in the context of safety guideline failures' 17.12.19

are starting to see, the advent of this technology includes increases in insomnia, tinnitus, headaches, inability to concentrate and fatigue.

He has further discerned as a consequence of 5G testing: UK 5G ambulance service suicides, cases of panic in cattle in the Netherlands, bizarre, aggressive behavior in cattle and sheep in Germany, birth defects in Germany and France and hundreds of birds dropping from the sky due to sudden cardiac arrest during three days of 5G testing in a park near Rotterdam. His list goes on and on to also include insect death and increases in fires in South Korea.

Smaller life forms like insects are more sensitive to this wireless microwave radiation. At the beginning of this century, car drivers started to realise that insects were no longer splattering onto their windscreens as they used to: they were gone. Small creatures vanish, as there are no longer insects for them to feed upon.

Here is one woman's view –

The 5G mm waves cause non-contagious illnesses, destroy the immune system, disrupt haemoglobin levels, and alter the air we breathe and the water we drink. Videos of people from around the world bear witness to telecom workers installing 5G antennaa and towers next to schools (which are unoccupied until Fall 2020), "non-essential" businesses (which are unoccupied), on residential buildings, in parks and recreational fields, and along the streets that line cities and suburbs…all done while people are "quarantined" behind locked doors.

The beginnings of sickness that is caused by chronic exposure to radiation, such as chronically being exposed to 5G mini-towers placed on residencies, sounds a lot like Coronavirus. According to *Medical News Today,* which outlines the general acceptance of what constitutes Radiation Sickness, the symptoms are set in stages. The initial stage of a sufferer of radiation poisoning will exhibit extreme flu-like symptoms with nausea, diarrhea, vomiting, chills, malaise, sore throat, coughing, wheezing, laboured breathing, and mucus build-up. These are eerily similar to the symptoms of Coronavirus, as listed on the CDC's website. Combine that with the lack of oxygen in the air due to the absorption of it at 60gigaHertz, and you can add permanent damage to the lungs with lesions and more nausea and vomiting to the list. (Askmarissa.com '5G Causes coronavirus', 12.2.20)

A sombre warning was given in 2018 by a group of 230 medics and scientists to the EU, who largely ignored it:

We, the undersigned scientists, recommend a moratorium on the roll-out of the fifth generation, 5G, until potential hazards for human health and the environment have been fully investigated by scientists independent from industry. 5G will substantially increase exposure to radio frequency electromagnetic fields (RF-EMF)… and has been proven to be harmful for humans and the environment.

Pig-ignorant British 'experts' on this topic could benefit from studying a statement put out by one of the above scientists, Dr Martin Pall, entitled: *5G: Great risk for EU, U.S. and International Health! Compelling Evidence for Eight Distinct Types of Great Harm* which began: 'We know that there is a massive literature, providing a high level of scientific certainty, for each of eight pathophysiological effects caused by non-thermal microwave frequency EMF exposures.' (PDF online) British experts maintain an ostrich-like posture on these matters which is unlikely to change anytime soon, not least because of legal ramifications: once an assurance is given that a safety threshold is OK, revising it downwards by quite a few orders of magnitude might well open up the possibility of lawsuits.

Trapped on a Boat

We all heard about the fate of the luxury cruise ship *Diamond Princess* that was put into quarantine, but less about how it was equipped with the very latest 5G electronic gear. Half a dozen huge spheres for receiving the newest WiFi (see image) were strangely prominent. It's perfectly safe, the experts said.

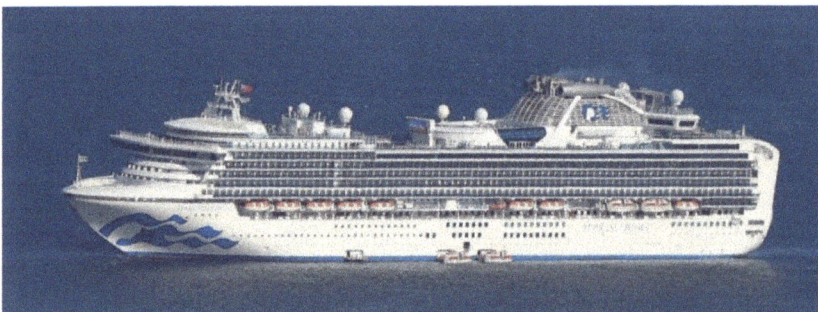

The satellite company involved announced that they were using a "hybrid medium earth orbit and geostationary network" so that these cruise ships could access the 'ground-breaking satellite-based communications system.' As part of a global 5G network, the satellite system works on 17-30 GHz. The lucky passengers were told, 'We offer the fastest WiFi on the high seas making it easier for you to stream movies' etc. Why, the ship had 75 miles of cable and 1,780 WiFi access points!

Did the passengers appreciate it? The ship became quarantined on February 3rd in a Japanese shipyard after a passenger had tested positive for C19. In the end, 381 passengers became sick and 14 died. Those illnesses and deaths were surely 5G casualties, as the passengers were trapped in a metal frame buzzing with powerful electrical frequencies from which they had no escape. That frequency, of tens of billions of cycles per second, seems to be perilous for life on earth.

There were about one thousand functioning artificial satellites circling the Earth in 2017 and that number has now doubled. Huge new fleets of satellites are being launched, to bring high-speed wireless internet to all corners of the Earth, and make video games even quicker. But, all of us are now in the position of the proverbial frog being boiled, as it fails to jump out of the pot while the temperature is slowly raised. She, Gaia, Mother Earth, the unique Emerald Sphere, is being mistreated and her creatures damaged.

The Change in Fifty Years

Before   **After**

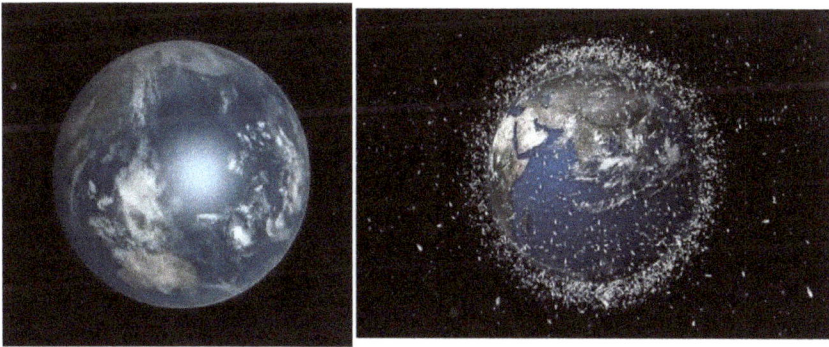

The magnetic field of the heart and the electric field of the brain are important in all sorts of subtle ways, and our feeling of well-being depends on them functioning properly. All of our nervous system is electrical. Creatures use very low-voltage electric fields and respond to magnetic fields optimally around that of Earth's intensity. Thus, wheat seeds will germinate better if aligned with the North-South magnetic field. This does unfortunately tend to be dismissed as 'crank' science. There is very little tradition in British science for magnetobiology or electrobiology, which are now becoming highly relevant.[57] When I used to look into this topic there would be rather little in English but there were Russian papers and

---

[57] The classic work on the topic is Alexandre Dubrov, *The Geomagnetic Field and Life*, 1978.

books to be consulted.

The Legal Challenge

Thank goodness that the group 'Legal Action Against 5G' (actionagainst5g.org/) is mounting a challenge against the immense new industries. It will be managed by the top British barrister Michael Mansfield QC.:

> 5G radiation will be sent from advanced antennas, in phased arrays, that transmit microwaves in narrow beams, a technology originally developed for military purposes. This will massively increase the exposure to radiation from those beams. Those beams will be nearly everywhere.

The problem here is that

> Industry has not produced a single study to show that 5G is safe or undertaken any risk assessment for effects on humans, wildlife and the environment for this laser-like beam forming technology.

That's certainly true. Moreover its 'safety levels' are absolutely bogus:

> Reassurance of safety is currently based on the long obsolete view point that radio frequency (RF) radiation can only cause harm above thermal, tissue heating, levels of exposure. This concept has been invalidated by hundreds of peer-reviewed published scientific papers.

For details of this see Appendix 3. It is surely the case that

> Nothing other than a legal challenge will force a government to take notice; this is the only way to ensure the government engages with the issue.
>
> We bring this case because we lack confidence in Public Health England.

Indeed! Anyone describing PHE as some kind of environmental protection agency can only be speaking in an ironic or Orwellian sense.

> The consequence of doing nothing will allow irreparable harm to all life, most particularly the unborn, children, the elderly, anyone with underlying health conditions and people with metal implants…Damage goes well beyond the human race, as there is growing evidence of harmful effects to both plants and animals.

Citizens need to endorse this brave campaign. Much of what people attribute to COVID-19 is actually being caused by the 5G rollout.

7

The Mandatory Vaccine

He [Gates] and other globalists are using it for mandatory vaccinations and microchipping people so we know if they've been tested. Over my dead body. Mandatory vaccinations? No way, Jose!
Roger Stone[58]

We're concerned here with the concept of a hoax, which we interpret as the unrolling of a *pre-ordained globalist agenda*. This is what has changed the world so quickly. Deeply prepared, it was activated at the key moment, which was the beginning of 2020. We will now attempt to sketch out the immensity of the agenda which is approaching as a forthcoming doom. Some kind of global surveillance society had been prepackaged and no-one could quite see how it would be implemented, until now, when it arrives with a vaccine.

Along with a DNA-modifying vaccine, citizens can anticipate receiving their *digital identity* 'ID2020' together with a *biometric immunity* passport. 'ID2020' has been well described as 'an electronic ID program that uses generalized vaccination as a platform for digital identity.'[59] It is worth meditating upon that definition. Evidently, the decision was finalised to roll it out in the year 2020 and that decision was made *before* the world had heard about C19. In January 29th, 2021 The Bundestag, Germany's parliament, ratified the implementation of 'Agenda ID 2020,' as being centralized electronic data collection on every citizen.

Here's some of the Chronology, which indicates how its

---

[58] Nypost.com Roger Stone: 'Bill Gates may have created coronavirus to microchip people' April 13
[59] Globalresearch.ca Peter Koenig, The Coronavirus COVID-19 Pandemic: The Real Danger is "Agenda ID2020"

unfolding *synchronized with* the C19 epidemic:

Sept 2019 Global Vaccination Summit in Brussels, to tackle causes of 'vaccine hesitancy.'

Sept. 2019 ID2020 Alliance summit held in New York to promote 'digital identity'

Oct. 2019 *Event 201* held at the John Hopkins University by Bill Gates et. al.

Nov. 2019 CEPI pledges $700m for development of DNA/RNA vaccines

Dec. 2020 Two-day Global Vaccine Safety Summit in Geneva by the WHO

Jan. 2020 CEPI announces initiation of programs to develop CV-19 vaccine

June 2020 UK hosts Global Vaccine Summit to promote GAVI, the Bill Gates' Vaccine alliance

(CEPI: Coalition for Epidemic Preparedness Innovations)

Genetic reporgamming

The 'Coalition for Epidemic Preparedness Innovations' was set up in 2107 at the Davos World Economic Forum. It brought together biotechnology and Big Pharma with the goal of global immunisation, using the new 'DNA/RNA vaccines.' But is this desirable? Numerous scientists have warned that once inside the cell nucleus, so-called 'messenger RNA' vaccines carry a risk of permanently changing a person's DNA in unpredictable ways. Damage could be inflicted upon future generations, with a vaccine which can adjust DNA ordering it to produce certain proteins.

Everywhere in this endeavour the tentacles of the Bill and Melinda Gates Foundation have been present, not least in the cofounding and funding of the CEPI. As James Corbett has noted, 'Every aspect of the current coronavirus pandemic involves organizations, groups and individuals with direct ties to Gates funding.' [60] Britain's Chief Medical Officer Chris Whitty was formerly on the CEPI advisory board and the UK government has donated £50 million to it while being advised by Whitty. Years earlier in 2008 he had received a grant from Gates to the tune of $40 million for malaria vaccination in Africa.[61]

In 2018, CEPI formed a partnership with Imperial College as we saw in Chapter 3, with the ambitious goal to "rapidly develop vaccines against pathogens — even unknown ones." In November 2019, CEPI committed $700 million to vaccine development, and that included "three vaccine platforms to develop vaccines against Disease X, a novel or unanticipated pathogen"' - that being the exact moment when the COVID infections seem to have begun. The UK government pledged £250 million to CEPI to help develop a C19 vaccine – the most that any country has given. Chris Whitty chairs the *UK Vaccine Network*, Boris Johnson has chaired a *Humanity Versus the Virus* conference and *Public Health England* is promoting the fatuous slogan 'Carry on vaccinating' (hashtag *#CarryOnVaccinating*). So there is a huge commitment of HMG to this kind of solution, which can sound benevolent until one appreciates the absence of choice that may be involved here, also its cumulative nature: children are going to be given more and more vaccines to 'protect' them, and what harm may this cause them?

It can sound benevolent if one is ignorant of the damage caused by vaccinations. Adverse effects caused by vaccines are common though not widely reported. For example, children used to be given the DTP vaccine (diphtheria, tetanus and perossis). A study of over a thousand children in Denver, Colorado, found after DTP that only

[60] James Corbett 'Part One: How Bill Gates Monopolized Global Health' 1 May
[61] Vanessa Beeley, 'COVID–19: The Big Pharma players behind UK Government lockdown' *UK Column* 6 May.

7% of those vaccinated were free from untoward reactions, which included pyrexia (53%), acute behavioral changes (82%), prolonged screaming (13%), and listlessness, anorexia and vomiting. 71% of those receiving second injections of DTP experienced two or more of the reactions monitored."[62] Here is a comment by Barbara Loe Fisher, of the private National Vaccine Information Center:

> How many children have [adverse] vaccine reactions every year? .. There have been estimates that perhaps less than 5 or 10 percent of doctors report hospitalizations, injuries, deaths, or other serious health problems following vaccination. The 1986 Vaccine Injury Act contained no legal sanctions for not reporting; doctors can refuse to report and suffer no consequences. Even so, each year about 12,000 reports are made to the Vaccine Adverse Event Reporting System [VAERS]; parents as well as doctors can make those reports.[63] However, if that number represents only 10 percent of what is actually occurring, then the actual number may be 120,000 vaccine-adverse events [per year]..[or] the real number may be 1.2 million vaccine-adverse events annually.[64]

C19 vaccine makers will be indemnified from financial liability no matter how many casualties they may cause. That is so wrong! They need to be fully responsible for such adverse reactions. The World Health Organisation had declared 'vaccine hesitancy' to be among the 'top ten threats to global health.' (January 2019) Then the CEO of YouTube has announced that it will be deleting any video deemed to be in contravention of advice being given by the WHO. These are very authoritarian steps.

Dire new legislation is appearing, as if the British Government is gearing up for a full-scale operation. Children in care-homes can now be forcibly vaccinated without parental consent and against

[62] Barker and Pichichero, *Lancet,* May 28, 1983, p. 1217
[63] RT Chen, B. Hibbs, 'Vaccine safety,' *Pediatric Annals,* July 1998: 445-458
[64] Tapnewswire.com 'One million adverse vaccine events go unreported annually' Tapestry, 21 May.

their expressed wish.[65] Persons returning on a plane flight to the UK can expect a 14-day quarantine, with enforcement officers liable to come a-knocking on your door to make sure you are in, or else you face a hefty fine.[66] And this applies to perfectly healthy people! These are deep violations of basic human rights.

Vaccination at Warp Speed

British Health Minister Matt Hancock has said he is looking 'very seriously' at making vaccination mandatory for state schools (*Guardian*, 29.9.19). Hancock owns the Porton Biopharma Ltd company in his capacity of Minister of Health. That was formed in June 2018, when 'Public Health England' transferred its drug development programs to it. Thus PHE will receive a dividend from any vaccines developed there. If it is profiting from vaccine sales it cannot be independent. Can a Minister of Health really owns a subsidiary of Britain's chief biological warfare unit?

Slowly, Bill Gates' 'digital identity' concept is being introduced. People are going to need a certificate, Matt Hancock has explained, to tell whether they have 'immunity', that is to say whether they have 'the antibodies' in their bloodstream and such certificates will permit them to 're-enter society.' Thus he stated,

'We're developing this critical science to know the impact of a positive antibody test and to develop the systems of certification to ensure people who have positive antibodies can be given assurances of what they can safely do.[67]

That echoes what Bill Gates declared at a 2015 TED talk: 'Eventually we will have some digital certificates to show who has recovered or been tested recently, or when we have a vaccine, who

---

[65] *Daily Mail*, 'Court of appeal says children in need can be vaccinated against their parent's wishes' 23.5
[66] *Mail* 23 May
[67] *Mail* 21 May, 'Immunity Certificates for people who have recovered from coronavirus…'

has received it.'

What 'immunity' means and how long it might last is far from clear. The UK government has not yet stated what as immunity certificate will be like - whether it will be tattooed under your skin, on your mobile phone or whatever. Ten million antibody tests have been ordered by HM government. Germany has similar plans but says the concept has first to be approved by the country's top ethicists!

We should here listen to the venerable science journal *Nature*. Its editorial has warned: 'In our view, any documentation that limits individual freedoms on the basis of biology risks becoming a platform for restricting human rights, increasing discrimination and threggatening - rather than protecting - public health.'[68]

'Your papers please' *Ihr papiere bitte!* was and maybe still is a Nazi trope, indicating an oppressive society, a cultural metaphor for life in a police state. Do we want that? It may become the new normal for documents to be required for travel or even to be allowed to shake hands with someone. The UK's Home Secretary has stated: 'I think we all recognise now that social distancing is here to stay,' a statement which indicates a powerful shared belief in the phantomic *Doom Virus*. Soon your mobile phone may track those with whom you come into contact and instruct you to self-isolate for fourteen days – without telling you where the alleged infection has come from!

This may be a good time to get rid of your mobile phone and go back to a simple landline, one which does not take messages.

On 23 April Gates stated: "the only way to return the world to where it was before COVID-19 showed up is a highly effective vaccine that prevents the disease." He alluded to 'Pandemic 1' as if this were the first of many to come, with 'Pandemic 2' as coming

---

[68] *Nature* editorial, 'Ten reasons why immunity passports are a bad idea.' 21 May.

next. That will enable him to start marketing his Mark-II vaccine, just like a new edition of his Microsoft programs. However getting everyone genetically modified will not return the world to its former condition, far from it. To achieve that desired goal, one would merely have to adjust the cause-of-death definition so that it no longer includes persons dying of various assorted conditions such as heart failure, old age etc. Then the death figures would drop like a stone and the perceived menace of C19 would fade away like a dream forgotten.

In May stock prices surged for the US biotech firm Moderna as it delivered its first results of the 'coronavirus vaccine.' A 'warp speed' timeline had been decreed by the US President, so the product was not tested on monkeys but was applied straightaway to human subjects. Only exceptionally healthy volunteers were allowed to participate in the test. Using an experimental mRNA technology it found *that twenty percent of the subjects became extremely ill*: 'three of the 15 human guinea pigs in the high dose cohort suffered a 'serious adverse event' within 43 days of receiving Moderna's jab' The effects were defined as 'preventing daily activity and requiring medical intervention.'[69]

Let us mull over the wise words of Joseph Mercola:

> Remember, government cannot keep you safe from disease. Only you can do that. Government really should safeguard public freedom, not public health at the expense of human liberty.[70]

A Medicine that works?

If anyone is worried about getting ill due to a coronavirus, there could be a cheap and effective antidote. It's an anti-malaria drug called chloroquinone. Government health advisors have been

---

[69] thetruthseeker.co.uk/?p=207598   Robert Kennedy, '20% of human subjects sustained severe injuries from Gates-Fauci coronavirus vaccine'
[70] J. Mercola, 'How Bill Gates Monopolised public health' Mercola.com 21 May

decrying its use, while advising a 'lockdown' until some vaccine is developed.

C19 is a coronavirus, labelled SARS-CoV-2 and while not exactly the same virus as SARS-CoV-1 it is genetically related. In 2005, the US *Virology Journal* published a major article entitled, "Chloroquine is a potent inhibitor of SARS coronavirus infection and spread." SARS (Severe Acute Respiratory Syndrome) is caused by coronavirus, and doctors were finding that taking that medicine together with zinc was an effective cure.

When the SARS outbreak hit the USA in 2003 – caused by a coronavirus dubbed SARS- CoV – the National Institute for Health concluded that chloroquinine was an effective antidote to that coronavirus. Both chloroquine and it's milder derivative hydroxychloroquine (HCQ) can be used for treating coronavirus and may also prevent future cases, i.e. they seem able **to** function both as a cure and a vaccine. They work best with a zinc supplement. Hydroxychloroquine is a decades old drug with a long safety record and a small price tag.

A safe, effective and cheap medicine is far from being what Big Pharma is seeking, and soon the fatwas went out. The Governor of New York banned the use of HCQ in the entire state on March 6 and the governors of Nevada and Michigan soon followed suit. By March 28 the whole country was under incarceration-in-place bans. In the UK, the Medical and Healthcare Regulatory Agency decreed that chloroquine and hydroxychloroquine should not be used to treat COVID-19 outside clinical trials, while NHS England has 'strongly discouraged' GPs from using these drugs for C19.

In France on January 13 the Minister of Health Agnes Buzyn classified chloroquine as a "poisonous substance" that would henceforth be available only by prescription – and this is a substance that had been sold off-the-shelf in France for half a century. Then in February the world-renowned infectious disease expert Professor

The Mandatory Vaccine

Didier Raoult, head of the Institut Hospitalo-Universitaire (IHU) Méditerranée Infection in Marseille, and a team of researchers reported that the use of hydroxychloroquine administered with both azithromycin and zinc cured 79 of 80 patients with only "rare and minor" adverse events. "In conclusion," these researchers wrote, "we confirm the efficacy of hydroxychloroquine associated with azithromycin in the treatment of COVID-19 and its potential effectiveness in the early impairment of contagiousness."[71]

The initial French lockdown came on March 17th, then on the 29th of March the LCI news channel revealed that entire the stock of chloroquine at the French central pharmacy has been *stolen*. Another French medic confirmed this, that 'The central pharmacy for the hospitals announced today that they were facing a total rupture of stocks, that they were pillaged.' It was all gone! Only one French company manufactured chloroquine, and it is under judicial investigation.

The New York physician Dr. Vladimir Zelenko reported on 23rd of March –the date of the UK lockdown - that he and his team had used a combination of HCQ, azithromycin, and zinc to successfully treat five hundred high-risk C19 patients. He reported "ZERO deaths, ZERO hospitalizations, and ZERO intubations [ventilator uses]" and "no serious negative side effects" caused by the drug protocol. He was interviewed by Rudi Giuliani who seemed to endorse his claims, and tweeted that Dr Zelenko had treated 699 'high-risk COVID-19 patients.' Zelenko stated that patients under 60 would be 'fine' and didn't need to worry, whereas C19 patients who were older or had a chronic medical condition he would treat immediately with the "cocktail."[72] His view of how it worked was:

---

[71] *Global Research* 'Why France Is Hiding a Cheap and Tested Virus Cure' by Pepe Escobar 27 March
[72] *American Spectator* George Perry, https://spectator.org/the-20-solution-to-coronavirus-anecdotal-evidence-is-a-life-saver/

98

> We know that hydroxychloroquine helps Zinc enter the cell. We know that zinc slows viral replication within the cell. Regarding the use of azithromycin, I am not sure. These three drugs are well known and usually well tolerated, hence the risk to the patient is low.

He reckoned that, compared to seasonal flu, COVID-19 was three times more contagious. If anyone wants to try this medicine I'd recommend taking careful note of the quantities he recommended because a wrong dose can be dangerous.

In May the US Department of Health and Human Services announced that Sandoz had donated 30 million doses of HCQ and Bayer one million doses of CQ to the Strategic National Stockpile. The US Health Service has assured that these drugs will be "distributed and prescribed by doctors to hospitalized teen and adult patients with COVID-19, as appropriate." Major US hospitals have started to publish COVID-19 treatment protocols that include the use of HCQ, as physicians are starting to use HCQ either alone or in combination with azithromycin to successfully treat COVID-19 patients.

If there is a disease caused by C19, then all along there could have been a fairly traditional remedy which does not need a lockdown or a vaccine or billions of dollars for healthcare.

Bogus science pushed by Big Pharma

This traditional medical remedy HCQ was damned by the *British Medical Association* in its journal *The Lancet*, on May 21st.[73] A large-scale study was featured, wherein its authors were 'unable to confirm a benefit of hydroxychloroquine or chloroquine.' Use of these medicines 'was associated with decreased in-hospital survival and an increased frequency of ventricular arrhythmias when used for treatment of COVID-19.' In other words they killed people. The

---

[73] The Lancet.com, Mandep Mehra *et.al.*,

report made global news and prompted the WHO to halt the hydroxychloroquine arm of its global trials.

On that same day a massive go-ahead for the new vaccine was announced. The Cambridge company AstraZeneca was awarded $1.2 billion by a US Biomedical fund. AstraZeneca operates in over a hundred countries so that millions have been using its medicines. This British firm, rather than the US Biotech giant Moderna, secured the big contract. It has undertaken to produce at least 400 million doses. It has a secure, total manufacturing capacity for one billion doses! Deliveries are scheduled to begin in September 2020.[74]

The vaccine itself is being developed by the University of Oxford, a 'recombinant adenovirus vaccine' by the University's Jenner Institute, working with the Oxford Vaccine Group. It contains the genetic material of SARS-CoV-2 spike protein, and is meant to trigger a strong immune response with just one dose. But will it work? The head of the Jenner Institute has stated in an interview that 'At the moment there's a 50% chance that we get no result at all' because they may not be able to find enough people who are going to catch the virus, to test whether their vaccine gives immunity.[75] Normally these programs take years to develop.

This is indeed Trump's 'Operation Warp Speed' program in action. It's a staggering commitment for an untested program that might not work, or might permanently damage human DNA. The two oldest British colleges are collaborating and Britons will be first to get access, if the vaccine is 'successful'. AstraZeniker has agreed to distribute 30 million doses to the U.K. in September, and a total of 100 million - which sounds like it's for everyone.

---

[74] Fiercepharma.com 'AstraZeneca scores $1.2B from U.S., signs up to deliver hundreds of millions of COVID-19 vaccines' 21 May

[75] https://www.rt.com/uk/489606-oxford-coronavirus-vaccine-50-percent-chance-success/

That *Lancet* killer-blow against the traditional medicine remedy also appeared in the prestigious *New England Journal of Medicine*. Normally, two medical journals would never publish the same paper at the same time and that indicates the powers that are involved here. The study claimed to be based upon a gigantic group of 96,000 patients suffering from COVID-19 in 671 hospitals from Australia. It was widely reported as showing that the CHQ medicine was a total failure - but then, a mere thirteen days later, *The Lancet* had to retract the article, on the grounds that no-one could find its data! A gifted undercover journalist (Celia Farber undercoverdc.com) exposed the whole fraud, and her implication was that the data had never existed. The data had supposedly been gathered by a company 'Surgisphere' whose employees featured a science fiction writer and an adult model. Two venerable medical-science journals have greatly damaged their credibility by publishing junk science.

It gets worse. At the time of publication, the Editor of *The Lancet* knew of the fraud! He was then attending what was supposedly a strictly secret 'closed door' Chatham House meeting, but his words have been leaked by a French source.[76] A Dr Douste-Blazy, formerly France's Health Minister and then Under-Secretary-General of the United Nations, has revealed how 'both the editors of the *Lancet* and the *New England Journal of Medicine* stated their concerns about the criminal pressures of Big Pharma on their publications.' The remarkable words of the Lancet's chief editor Horton were:

> Now we are not going to be able to, basically, if this continues, publish any more clinical research data, because the pharmaceutical companies are so financially powerful today and are able to use such methodologies, as to have us accept papers which are apparently methodologically

[76] Brighteon.com, "Hydroxychloroquine Lancet Study: Former France Health Minister blows the whistle"

perfect but which, in reality, manage to conclude what they want to conclude… This is very, very serious!"[77]

Can the *Lancet* recover from this scandal? In whom can one trust? Can the scientific method still work? One thing's for sure: the medical profession is in danger of drifting a very long way away from its sacred, primary axiom: 'First, do no harm.'

A tweet summed up the debacle:

Sean Da... @seanm... ✓

The entire study was fake. Congratulations on using garbage science from con artists to scare sick people away from potentially life-saving treatment. Hope the dank anti-Trump burns were worth it. https://twitter.com/julianborger/status/1263819256682237953 ...

Julian Bor... @julianbor... ✓

Trump on hydroxychloroquine, April 4: "What do you have to lose? Take it."

The Lancet: https://twitter.com/EricTopol/status/1263811764287725574 ...

6,159 2:33 PM - Jun 4, 2020 Twitter
Ads
2,955 people are talking about this
and

Asymptomatic persons not infectious

The biggest lie by far is that of asymptomatic transmission. Indeed, it may one day become known as the biggest lie, told to the largest number of people, in the shortest space of time - Rob Slane

---

[77] naturalnews.com, 'Leaked conversation of Lancet and NEJM Editors-In-Chief reveals they already know Big Pharma ...' 10 June. Hear Dr Simone Gold telling this *Lancet* story, in her talk (Bitchute), 'The truth about the covid-19 Vaccine' 14.1.21 at 20 mins.

On June 6th a WHO spokesperson said that people who showed no symptoms – and that is nearly everybody – were not infectious, i.e. they could not normally transmit the disease: "From the data we have, it still seems to be rare that an asymptomatic person actually transmits onward to a secondary individual. It's very rare" (Dr. Maria Van Kerkhove, head of WHO's emerging diseases and zoonosis unit at a news briefing from the UN agency's headquarters at Geneva). Clearly that would negate the entire rationale of lockdown and social distancing. It implies rather that one should isolate only persons who actually had the disease - but that would take us back into the normal, traditional medical practice and no pharmaceutical companies are going to make hundreds of billions of dollars if that view were to prevail. She was quickly pressured to backpedal: no, she hadn't actually meant that. But, as if not realising the huge implications, of bringing down the whole house of cards, she did say it.[78]

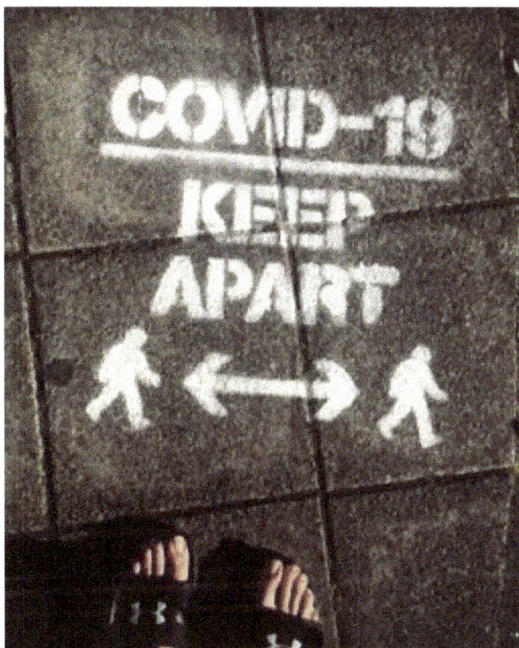

---

[78] Mike Adams, Natural news, 'The WHO just obliterated every argument for mandatory vaccines…' 8.6.20

8

2020: there was No Pandemic[79]

2020 saw 14% more deaths than average, last year in England & Wales and that amounted to seventy-five thousand extra deaths. We here use the Office of National statistics figures, as it gives total weekly deaths, and it also gives an average value of corresponding weekly deaths over the previous five years.[1]

That compares with the figure of ninety thousand deaths for the entire United Kingdom that year, due allegedly to covid-19.

We here ask and answer the question, what caused that excess of deaths? The answer will not be certain, but will be the simplest possible explanation. By Occam's razor we are obliged to take it.

For the first quarter of last year, deaths in England and Wales were down: for whatever reason, overall weekly mortality was 3% below the yearly average. Then around the spring equinox on March 23rd Lockdown was announced and suddenly, deaths surged right up so that thousands of extra deaths started happening week after week. That continued all through April and May and then finally, in the first week of June Britons were allowed out again: with relief we could walk the streets and parks, cafes and pubs opened up again.

Those months of Lockdown saw fifty-nine thousand excess

---

[79] For URL links, see article 'There is no Pandemic' published in Unz.com (NB it had six hundred comments).

deaths, see graph. (That comes from counting the eleven weeks ending 27 March to the 5th June, as being the lockdown period.)The question arises as to what caused them? Could it have been, for example, the shock? The month of April averaged ninety percent more deaths than usual! Then May was not quite so bad, as folk got used to the grim new reality.

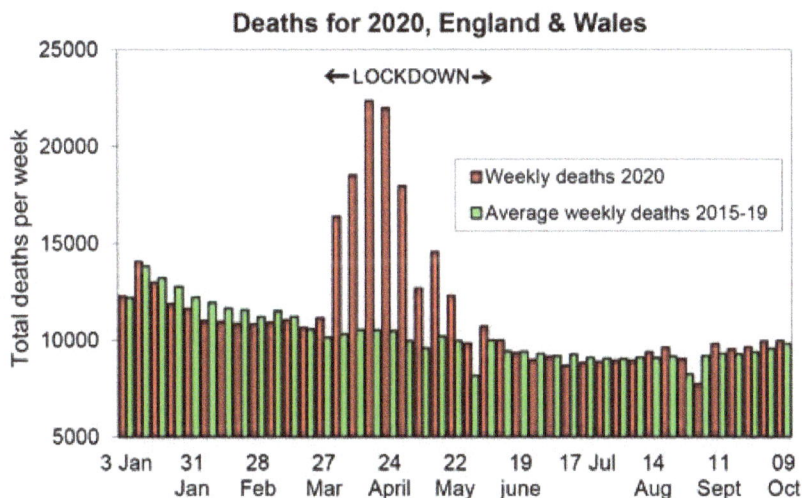

Deaths for 2020, England & Wales

Figure: weekly data from the Office of National Statistics for 2020, comparing total mortality per week with its estimated average from the previous five years.

In the weeks after the Lockdown i.e. after the first week of June the whole excess of deaths suddenly vanished. Over the next four months deaths remained exactly average compared to previous years.

The graph shows this distinct, three-stage process.

Total deaths data for weeks ending –

2020 / 2015-19 average

12 wks 3 Jan–20 Mar,   138,916 / 143,738 = – 4,822 => -3%

11 wks 27 Mar– 5 Jun, 168,396 / 109,703 = 58,693 => 54%

18 wks 12 Jun – 9 Oct, 166,392 / 165,808 = 584   => 0%

105

These figures suggest that it is the lockdown itself and not any virus, that caused the excess deaths.

We're here reminded of a careful survey done last May which found that, in all countries with reliable death-figures, their increase in mortality began after the lockdown was imposed and not before. There is a simple difference between cause and effect: the cause comes first, before the effect!

A second Lockdown was imposed over the month of November. This lacked the same terror and shock value of the first and so only reached a net 18% excess of mortality: for the five weeks from week ending 6 November to that of 4th December there were nine thousand excess deaths, compared to the seasonal average.

After the autumn equinox as the nights grew longer the government again started to terrorise the population with talk of the 'dark winter' to come. Somehow they knew that a 'second wave' was coming, and so there would have to be a 'second lockdown' and no Christmas. Here's what I predicted in a podcast on 20th October:

They are trying to resuscitate another big scare, trying to claim there is a second wave ... come this autumn, they have started drumming up fear again, they have imposed these levels of Lockdown which are rather terrifying. A lot of stress they are putting on people, I've been wondering, are the deaths going to go up again like last time?

Did that happen? The figures show as before a surge around the time of the lockdown and just before it, however this time it did not vanish after the lockdown. That's because there was not really any easing up. On the contrary yet more draconian measures were announced, with the unheard-of measure of police stopping people walking outdoors, to ask them if they had good reason to be out of their house? Meeting friends was forbidden, etc. That pressure pushed up the mortality even more and we here especially note the 'Christmas week' ending 25th December, with a whopping 45% excess mortality! That is not a merry Christmas, it's an extra three and a half thousand people popping off (as compared to previous years) in a week, caused presumably by shock and despair of Xmas being cancelled. The week after that it was still very high, 26% excess, as folk faced the bleak new year.

It helps to express that excess mortality as overall monthly means, for the last few months of 2020. Thus taking each month as a whole and selecting four weeks of data for each month:

September from weeks ending 11 Sept to 2 Oct.	+4%
October	9 Oct to 30th Oct	+7%
November	6 Nov to 27 Nov	+18%
December	4 Dec to 1st Jan	+21%

Slowly the excess deaths (comparing, as before, with previous years) have increased through the autumn and winter. The month of December had ten thousand extra deaths. Should one take the government's view, that these deaths were caused by the CV19 virus, and that the increasingly severe restrictions were a necessary response to 'contain' the spread of this virus? A simpler hypothesis would be that there is no virus killing people, whereas the stress of bankruptcy, solitude, loneliness, etc. imposed by government edicts really has been killing people. Thus for example 'tier 4' was announced on 19th December for large parts of England and that resulted in the highest mortality for the week following. That knockout blow to everyone's Christmas – never banned since the days of Oliver Cromwell – had the deep impact, driving up the mortality index.

Overall it would appear to be the government's lockdown policy that has been killing people and not some new disease. Stress, loneliness, fear and despair have been causing the excess of deaths: together with emptying out of hospitals, especially of old folk and cancellation of normal services because of the 'pandemic.' If the government knows this, then it is a population-reduction program.

A recent US Centre for Disease Control report agreed with the approach we've here taken, that the significance of CV19 can only be appreciated in terms of total mortality. Published on the John Hopkins University website on 22nd November (but soon removed), it endorses the view that no virus is killing people, any more than normal flu, whereas deaths from other causes are being re-classified as Covid19:

According to new data, the U.S. currently ranks first in total COVID-19 cases, new cases per day and deaths. Genevieve Briand, assistant program director of the Applied Economics master's degree program at Hopkins, critically analyzed the effect of COVID-19 on U.S. deaths using data from the Centers for Disease Control and Prevention (CDC) in her webinar titled "COVID-19 Deaths: A Look at U.S. Data."

From mid-March to mid-September, U.S. total deaths have reached 1.7 million, of which 200,000, or 12% of total deaths, are COVID-19-related. Instead of looking directly at COVID-19 deaths, Briand focused on total deaths per age group and per cause of death in the U.S. and used this information to shed light on the effects of COVID-19.

She explained that the significance of COVID-19 on U.S. deaths can be fully understood only through comparison to the number of total deaths in the United States.

After retrieving data on the CDC website, Briand compiled a graph representing percentages of total deaths per age category from early February to early September, which includes the period from before COVID-19 was detected in the U.S. to after infection rates soared.

Surprisingly, the deaths of older people stayed the same before and after COVID-19. Since COVID-19 mainly affects the elderly, experts expected an increase in the percentage of deaths in older age groups. However, this increase is not seen from the CDC data. In fact, the percentages of deaths among all age groups remain relatively the same.

"The reason we have a higher number of reported COVID-19 deaths among older individuals than younger individuals is simply because every day in the U.S. older individuals die in higher numbers than younger individuals," Briand said.

Briand also noted that 50,000 to 70,000 deaths are seen both before and after COVID-19, indicating that this number of deaths was normal long before COVID-19 emerged. Therefore, according to Briand, not only has COVID-19 had no effect on the percentage of deaths of older people, but it has also not increased the total number of deaths.

These data analyses suggest that in contrast to most people's assumptions, the number of deaths by COVID-19 is not alarming. In fact, it has relatively no effect on deaths in the United States...

When Briand looked at the 2020 data during that seasonal period, COVID-19-related deaths exceeded deaths from heart diseases. This was highly unusual since heart disease has always prevailed as the leading cause of deaths. However, when taking a closer look at the death numbers, she noted something strange. As Briand compared the number of deaths per cause during that period in 2020 to 2018, she noticed that instead of the expected drastic increase across all causes, there was a significant decrease in deaths due to heart disease. Even more surprising, as seen in the graph below, this sudden decline in deaths is observed for all other causes.

This trend is completely contrary to the pattern observed in all previous years. Interestingly, as depicted in the table below, the total decrease in deaths by other causes almost exactly equals the increase in deaths by COVID-19. This suggests, according to Briand, that the COVID-19 death toll is misleading. Briand believes that deaths due to heart diseases, respiratory diseases, influenza and pneumonia may instead be recategorized as being due to COVID-19.

Based on this analysis, the best way to end the ongoing mass-killing of elderly Britons would be to terminate the lockdowns and resume normal life. As Dr Simone Gold (of Frontline Doctors) well explained, CV19 is just 'killing' elderly people who were about to die anyhow. It cannot be shown that 'having' CV19 i.e. testing PCR-'positive' contributed to shortening their life. So that isn't a causal connection, i.e. the alleged illness has not 'caused' their death. That's why the age-distribution of CV-19 is indistinguishable from that of the normal population.

The average age of death in England & Wales is 81.5 years, while the average age of 'Covid-19 fatalities' is 82.4 years (ONS data). What this tells us is very simple: the disease does not exist.

The concept of PCR 'testing' has always been fraudulent. The so-called PCR 'test' multiplies up fragments of nucleotide-chains and the number of 'positive' cases depends on the multiplication factor used as well as how many persons are tested. There will never come a time when the virus is 'cured' or 'solved' or whatever people imagine the government is trying to do (if it knows!), such that the PCR test ceases to generate 'positive' tests. No-one will ever give you evidence that people who test 'positive' get ill more often than others. Is there an aim of government policy, aside from terrorising the populace? Is it to kill the virus? That can never happen because the virus isn't alive.

The World Health Organization has now backtracked over the PCR 'test', saying (January 13th) it is merely a diagnostic tool that can assist. It now advises –

> Where test results do not correspond with the clinical presentation, a new specimen should be taken and retested using the same or different NAT technology.

In other words, a single PCR test should not be used for diagnosing Sars-Cov-2 infection. It's merely a guide!

Most PCR assays are indicated as an aid for diagnosis, therefore, health care providers must consider any result in combination with timing of sampling, specimen type, assay specifics, clinical observations, patient history, confirmed status of any contacts, and epidemiological information.

So we finally have it that the PCR cannot be relied upon a diagnostic test. Which is exactly what its inventor Kary Mullis said. So forget all of the figures you've heard about 'cases' and 'covid deaths' – they cannot be relied upon.

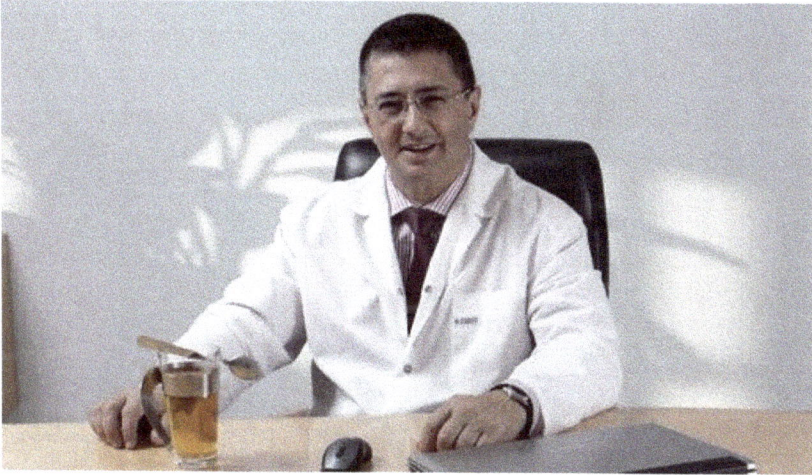

If one did want to believe there was a disease associated with this virus, then surely we'd agree with Dr Alexander Myasnikov, appointed last year as Russia's chief medical advisor. In an interview he explained how the world had greatly over-reacted to the CV19 story and death numbers in the West were greatly over-counted. He added:

> It's all exaggerated. It's an acute respiratory disease with minimal mortality.

Thus the former Chief Medical Officer of Ontario has recently challenged his government's policy saying, "We're Being Locked-down for an Infection Fatality Rate of Less than 0.2%?" and the lockdown is not "supported by strong science." He here means, that for those who test PCR-positive one in five hundred will die. The time-period here involved needs to be defined, eg it could be one month: we all die, and given the median age of alleged-CV19 deaths is around 80 that could well be a normal rate of mortality –

especially if they are PCR-testing everyone admitted to hospitals.

Last November a Cornish nurse went public, saying the hospital wards had been empty over months when it was claimed they were overflowing. She said whenever they had flu patients they were classified as Covid: 'flu and Covid cases are now recorded as 'the same thing' on death certificates.' That wouldn't be necessary if the disease really existed. Not surprisingly, the flu this winter has mysteriously vanished. One woman who walked round her local hospital filming its empty wards was arrested by police entering her home the next day.

The virus itself cannot be shown to exist, by which we mean that it cannot be reliably differentiated from all the other normal coronaviruses, that have been with us since time began. It has never been isolated, let's be clear about that. Last April an EU science department admitted:

> No virus isolates with a quantified amount of the SARS-CoV-2 are currently available ...

And the same thing was echoed a few months later by the US Centre for Disease Control:

> Since no quantified virus isolates of the 2019-nCoV are currently available, assays [diagnostic tests] designed for detection of the 2019-nCoV RNA were tested with characterized stocks of in vitro transcribed full length RNA...[2]

In other words, nobody can hold a test-tube or petri-dish and say, 'Here is COVID-19.' Published gene-sequences of the alleged virus are mere hypothetic constructs. Yes some disease broke out in Wuhan in November 2019 and yes the Chinese authorities published a gene-sequence allegedly of it, but so what?

Fear Porn Promotion

The government needs your fear. It wants your attention but knows that it has no prospect of improving your life in any way. Thus we have a health minister who knows nothing about health or well-being: he can get your attention by telling you that you won't be able to fly without a vaccine. They need your fear, and in the last century the government was able to arouse your fear by threatening to press the nuclear button. That doesn't work any more. The UK govts latest exercise in fear-porn advises citizens to behave as if they are ill! ('Act like you've got it') Yes, that sounds just like how to promote health.

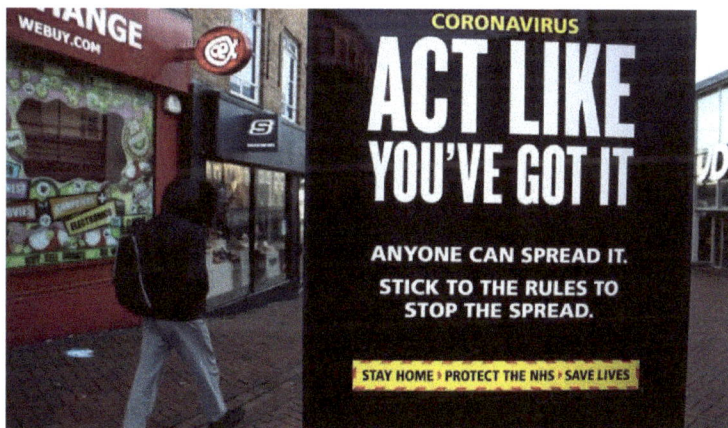

It further promotes the diabolical idea that perfectly healthy persons can transmit disease ('anyone can spread it'). Here one could quote the WHO expert Dr Maria van Kerkhove: 'From the data we have, it still seems to be rare that an asymptomatic person actually transmits onwards to a secondary individual. Its very rare.' (Head of the WHO Emerging disease and zoonosis unit at a news briefing from the UN agency's headquarters at Geneva, 6.6.20). Admittedly she was pressured to backpedal and retract, but she did say it.[3]

In the words of the *Daily Mail*, 'Terrifying new TV ads' are being promoted by the Government (23 Jan 2021) The above fear-porn promotion is through the US media agency Omnigov, who signed a £110 million Lockdown advertising deal – on March 2nd, three weeks *before* the Lockdown.

www.telegraph.co.uk › business › 2020/10/25 › govern... ▾

Government struck £119m Covid advertising deal weeks ...

Oct 25, 2020 — Ministers struck a deal worth up to **£119m** with one of the world's ... a
subsidiary of US ad titan **Omnicom**, on March 2 - the same day Prime ...

The journalist Neil Clark commented[4] on 'the report in
the Daily Telegraph newspaper that the UK government struck a
deal worth £119m with an American advertising company, OMD
Group, urging people to 'Stay Home, Stay Safe' a full three weeks
before Boris Johnson ordered a lockdown. Think about what this
means.' That meme 'Stay home Stay safe' would have been
blueprinted the previous year at the US 'Event 201' by Bill Gates et.
al. Fear blocks out rational, coherent thought which is why the
government needs it.

People may be forgetting how debilitating winter flu can be and how
it can last for weeks. Now they want to call it COVID. Let's here
support Prof. Dolores Cahill, who has been looking at the
sequencing of PCR testing. In Ireland it was found that of fifteen
hundred PCR tests 'all of them were influenza A and B, not one of
them were SARS-COV2.' Her group will be seeking legal action
where the tests come back as influenza rather than the specific CV19
and doctors can be sued for medical negligence. (Corbett Report, 23
mins) That sounds like a promising way of dealing with this
phantomic virus.

'Is this an epidemic of despair?' asked that perceptive
commentator Peter Hitchins. Scientists are trained not to take notice
of emotions and instead to look for material things as causative
agents, whereas here we agree with Peter Hitchens that the negative
soul-conditions of the populace caused by government policies are
leading to death. Hitchens' article quotes the distinguished
professor of medical microbiology, Sucharit Bhakdi. He said that
older people had the right to make efforts to stay fit, active, busy and
healthy. But he warned that the shutdown of society would
condemn them to early death by preventing this:

Social contacts and social events, theatre and music, travel and holiday recreation, sports and hobbies, all help to prolong their stay on earth. The life expectancy of millions is being shortened.

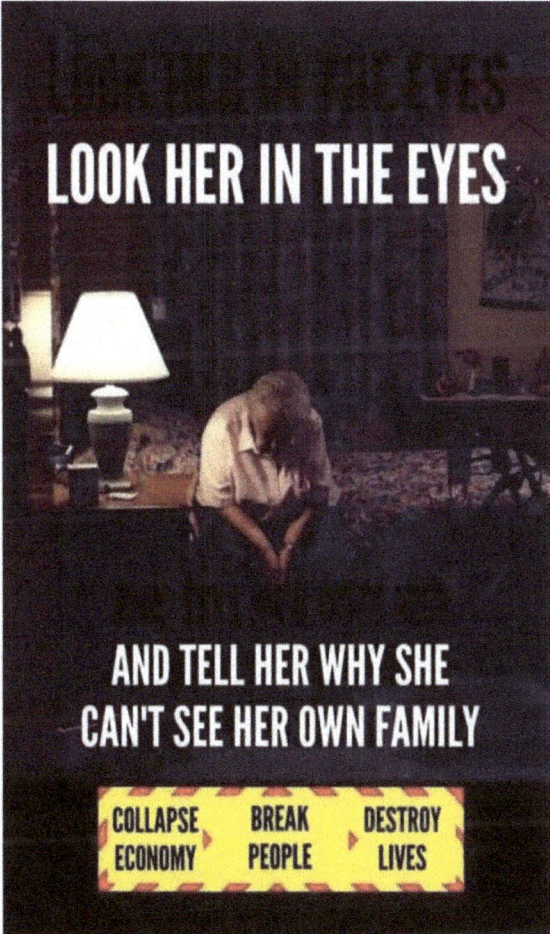

In a prediction that has turned out to be terribly accurate, he added: 'The horrifying impact on the world economy threatens the existence of countless people. The consequences for medical care are profound. Already services to patients who are in need are reduced, operations cancelled, practices empty, hospital personnel dwindling. All this will impact profoundly on our whole society.'

For comparison here is a graph showing the US weekly mortality rate over 2020. We see the very same effect, with a deficit in mortality in the first months of the year, followed by the huge excess in April right after Lockdown. This graph shows in red an excess of 280k deaths above normal-expected levels, following the lockdown. The web-page hosting this graph states 'The large spike in deaths in April 2020 corresponds to the coronavirus outbreak' but we here take a different view.

Excess deaths in the US in 2020

At the start of the year, the number of actual deaths was below the maximum amount predicted in statistical models based on historical data. But by the end of March, weekly deaths exceeded that upper threshold for predicted deaths. To date, **excess deaths** peaked in April.

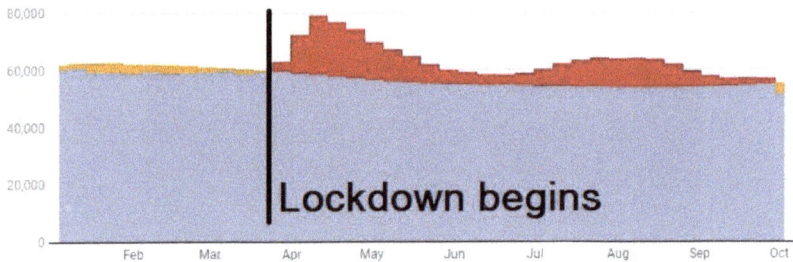

Data as of week ending Oct. 3, 2020 – released by CDC on Oct. 14, 2020.
Chart: The Conversation, CC-BY-ND · Source: CDC National Center for Health Statistics · Get the data

By way of contrast, Sweden had no lockdown, and so Swedish deaths right through 2020 remained absolutely normal [5]. They had no excess mortality that year! What that demonstrates is very simple – there is no pandemic.

[1] Using fifty-two weeks i.e. 364 days of the year, from the week ending 3rd January 2020 to that of 1st January 2021. The ONS helpfully compares each week in 2020 with an average value of that week for 2015-9. To see data, click on the Excel spreadsheet, let it download, open it up & click on '2020 data.'

[2] CDC '2019-Novel Coronavirus Real-Time PCR Diagnostic Panel performance characteristics' p.39, 13.7.20. This has been scrubbed from the Web, but see BMJ response to it.

[3] A huge Chinese study of ten million around Wuhan between May and June showed 'no evidence that positive cases without symptoms spread the disease': Nature 20.11.20 'Post-lockdown SARS-CoV-2 nucleic acid screening'.

[4] RT 'Covid-19 reverse psychology' by Neil Clarke, 28.10.20, deleted but

preserved on the Hugo Talks video

[5] hippy-end.livejournal.com/3918359.html   Click 'Google Translate'.

For URL references in this article, see online article 'There is no Pandemic' at Unz.com by the author N.B., this article obtained over six hundred comments.

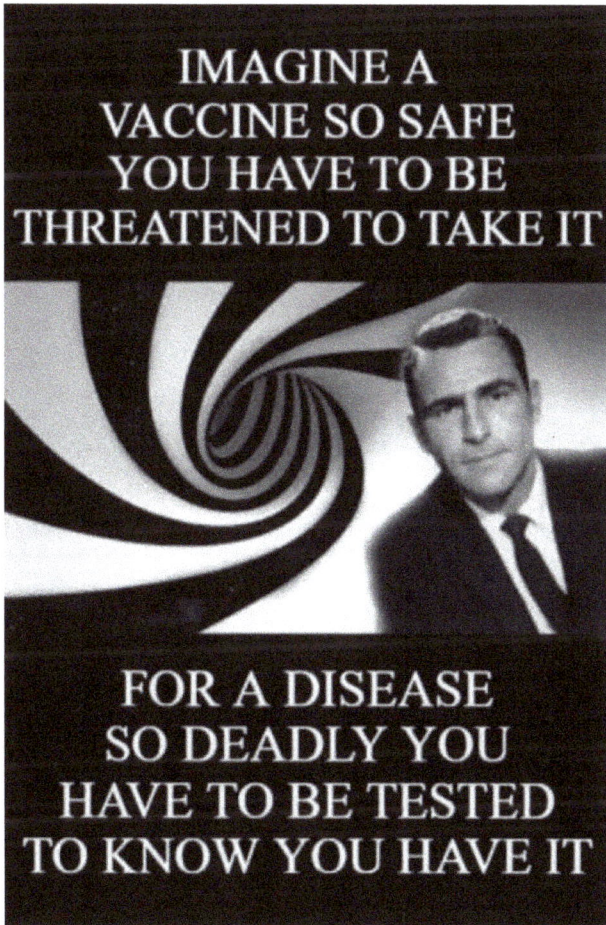

IMAGINE A VACCINE SO SAFE YOU HAVE TO BE THREATENED TO TAKE IT

FOR A DISEASE SO DEADLY YOU HAVE TO BE TESTED TO KNOW YOU HAVE IT

9

mRNA: is it a 'Vaccine'?

These "gene editing" vaccines are not medicine, they are a strange and menacing hybrid cocktail that was created to achieve an elusive political objective of which we still know very little.[80]

Lockdown Lunacy

The data is in: lockdowns serve no useful purpose and cause catastrophic societal and economic harms. They must never be repeated in this country.

Many international studies bear out that lockdowns have proven to be a complete failure as a public health measure to contain a respiratory virus. They did not succeed in their primary objective of containing spread yet have caused great harm.

- Hartgroup.org (a group of highly qualified UK doctors and scientists), 'Covid-19 an Overview of the Evidence' 18.3.21.

Right through January of 2021, UK citizens were imprisoned by means of what was really the strictest lockdown in the world and were *not allowed to step outside their own front door* unless they had some approved reason, eg buying food. Folks were arrested for standing on a street corner and it was illegal for people to open their own business if the authorities had not deemed them to be essential, it was illegal to leave the country unless for a reason the authorities have deemed as essential and even illegal to protest against any of the above policies.

In consequence we saw a huge peak in mortality in January. There were presumably two causes of this: the vaccine, and the enormous

---

[80] Globalresearch.co Mike Whitney 8.3.21, '*Vaccine Diabolos* and the Impending Wave of rare Neurodegenerative disorders.'

stress of a punitive lockdown, which seemed to have no end in sight. With spring starting to arrive in February things got better as the above bar-chart shows.

There have been four countries with far less restrictive lockdowns than other nations: Sweden, Japan, Belarus and Nicaragua, and these nations have been much criticized for that policy. In these four 'non-lockdowns' countries, the death rate ascribed to CV19 has been on average 239 per million of population. Five countries having the strictest lockdowns are the UK, the USA, France, Italy and Spain. On average their totals of 'covid deaths' were 1572 per million. That is six times higher.

Here are tables showing these results. Total scores are counted from the start of the pandemic in February up to March 1st of the next.[81] First, the selected high-stringency lockdown nations -

Strict Lockdown countries: Covid deaths per million

	Tot. deaths s Pop^n in millons
UK	123,125 / 66.5 => 1851
USA	527,394 / 328 => 1607
France	86,890 / 67.0 => 1296
Italy	97,945 / 60.3 => 1624
Spain	69,609 / 46.9 => 1484
Mean	deaths /m 1572

Little or no Lockdown countries: Covid deaths per million

Sweden	13,021/10.2 => 1276
Japan	7887 / 126 => 62
Belarus	1986 / 9.5 => 209
Nicarag.	173 / 6.5 => 26
Mean	Deaths /m 239

[81] Figures taken from www.worldometers.info/coronavirus/, at start of March: alethonews.com 'Believing in impossible things—and COVID19' 6.3.21 Dr Malcolm Kendrick

It will not escape the reader's notice that the ethically-damned 'no lockdown' group has a mortality rate *six times lower* than the strict-lockdown countries. This points to something catastrophically wrong with the reality-concepts here involved.

That is a staggering differential, and maybe people should talk about it, just a bit. How come no media, politicians or medical 'experts' ever discuss this differential? Have you ever heard anyone discuss it? Surely it is the most fundamental thing we know about the covid-19 'disease:' that 'it' kills people more, the stricter the lockdown.

There may be only two things we really know about this phantomic modern disease: the one as mentioned, that lockdown somehow enhances it; while the other pertains to the question, as to what a ward full of CV19 patients have in common? It is after all so very varied in its symptoms. An answer to this was given rather briefly by Dr Lee Merritt, that an Indonesian study had ascertained, wards full of Covid patients were found to be vitamin-D deficient.[82] That is the sunshine vitamin which the body cannot synthesise, and during this Lockdown we are probably all short of it.

Earlier chapters concluded that the more severe the lockdown, the more 'cases' appear, whereas here that difference is appearing far, far larger. The latter may be a fraudulent concept, however using it this huge differential appears. The effect here appears as greatly magnified from what earlier surveys have shown.

How come Britain is at or near the top of the list, and has remained so throughout this entire *faux*-pandemic? It is surely enjoying a higher level of collective psychotic derangement, *centred upon* a virus which does not really exist. It seems to me that the book written by Boris Johnson's father *The Virus* may be very relevant here, with its prescient, population-culling theme. Published in 1982, it concerned a mandatory vaccination program! It could account for

---

[82] https://sonsoflibertymedia.com/dr-lee-merit-the-vaxx-is-preparing-world-for-mass-death-event-video/ at 17 mins.

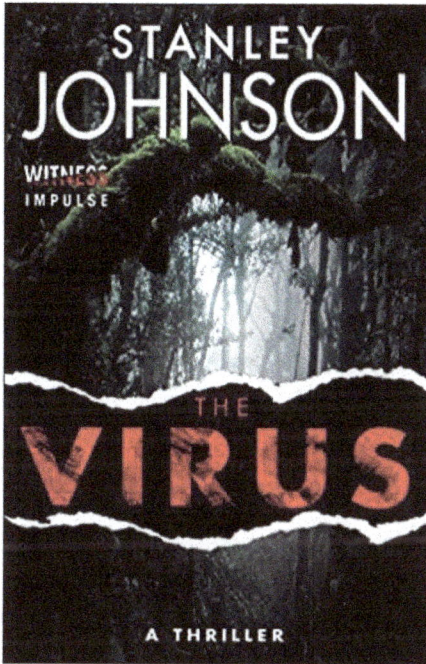

the Prime Minister's zombie-like certainty with which he utters each new hope-crushing, public-health-wrecking edict. The British people are now allegedly in a condition where a *majority* of them favor vax-passports to enter a gym or pub.

For example, through February he was dropping hints about a route map back to re-opening and some semblance of normality. Lots of very cheap air-flights were being advertised. Then suddenly at th4e spring equinox – like some dire echo of what happened a year ago, he announced that as from April 1st, no-one could fly out of the country unless they had a 'reasonable excuse.' What kind of language is that? Can you imagine airport officials asking people queuing up for tickets if they have a 'reasonable excuse' for wanting to fly?

So, what is the answer? I personally favour simple science-type experiments, but these are not going to happen! For example, hospitals tell us they have rooms full of Covid-19 patients. Could we just take samples of sputum from such patients and give them to healthy individuals? I will wager a large sum of money that no transmission of any disease thereby takes place.

But no, that can't happen, it's too simple. Okay, let's take a group of persons who have been 'vaccinated.' Simply give them the PCR test, quite apart from any questions of what the test may or may not measure. Do these persons test positive any less frequently than persons not vaccinated? Again, this is far too simple, no-one will do it. Again, I would wager a large sum of money that no difference would be found.

Let me suggest one last, final test – using the very old-fashioned idea of a scientific experiment, which can establish what is happening. I should apologise in advance for its embarrassing simplicity. The media blitz is continually telling us that fast vaccination of the populace is necessary to 'save lives.' Hurry, less people will die, if we're all vaccinated! I suggest *au contraire* that *more* people will thereby die i.e. that the policy is *causing* deaths not *preventing* them. Nothing could be simpler than discerning which of these two hypotheses is correct, by merely making available the death-statistics, separated into age-cohorts, of the two groups vacccinated versus non-vaccinated. Can the ONS not do this? We may be confident of the answer here.

Ideally one would like to see the mortality data divided into groups according to the 'vaccine' taken: AstroZenica, Pfitzer or Moderna, and thereby assess their different levels of lethality over the years. It would be a shame not to record this interesting consequence, of the huge experiment. In the words of Dr Joseph Mercola:

> If early statistics are any indication, we are facing the greatest public health calamity in modern history. No, I'm not talking about a third, fourth or fifth wave of COVID-19. I'm talking about the current vaccination campaign. I have no doubt that deaths caused by COVID-19 vaccines will end up far exceeding the number of actual COVID-19 deaths.[83]

We'll soon find out. Of one thing we may be very sure – if such delayed effects do start to kick in, they will be blamed upon some 'new wave' of the virus. Mercola added, 'Those ending up with permanent disability as a result of these vaccines will be at increased risk of early death.'

---

[83] Articles.mercola.com 'COVID-19 Vaccine Tested on Babies Even as Death Toll Mounts' 23.3.21

The Oxford-produced AstraZenica seems to be the most dangerous of the UK 'vaccines' According to a March 2, 2021, report, U.K. data show the AstraZeneca vaccine actually has 77% more adverse events and 25% more deaths than the Pfizer vaccine.[84] In March, more than 20 European countries suspended their use of AstraZeneca's vaccine following reports of deadly blood clots. The *Daily Mail* alluded to the 56-page report on strange illnesses and adverse effects following the Astrazenica jab. Merely entitled 'All UK spontaneous reports received between 4/01/21 and 07/03/21 for COVID-19 vaccine Oxford University/AstraZeneca,' it is certainly a frightening list of recorded harm. One is startled that people will queue up to take something with so long a published list of harmful effects.

2. Don't take the Jab

To quote the very quotable Sherry Tenpenny:

> Never before have so many companies tested so many different vaccines at the same time, against a virus that has not been isolated.

It's too soon to say what effect the several UK vaccines will have - Moderna, Astrozenica and Pfizer. One can however say for sure that they will *not* confer health benefits: the benefits they confer are civilian, such as permission to travel, go to work, to school, etc.

Nor are they vaccines in any traditional sense. A 'vaccine' has always meant an *attenuated pathogen,* which the organism is able to receive in a weakened form and thereby create antibodies to it, whereby a resistance to the disease is conferred. Moderna's product is an *experimental messenger-RNA platform* (modified RNA => 'Moderna'). No-one knows quite what it will do, which is why the manufacturers have legally indemnified themselves against any consequences. A vast experiment has begun, where taking the jab is

---

[84] *The Defender, Children's Health Defence*: 'UK data shows 402 reports of deaths following COVID vaccines' 3.2.21 by John Stone.

only the beginning: 'mRNA' has the curious ability to enter the cellular machinery of reproduction and duplicate itself, and after several months or maybe a year, what happens then? This substance will *not* flush out of your system, very much the contrary. It then has the ability to manufacture proteins and amino acids, which the body's immune system could well perceive as being foreign agents.

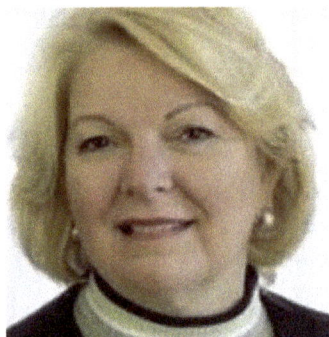

Figure: expert virologist Dr Sherry Tenpenny

And, what is the point? Why have a vaccine for an alleged illness that has so tiny a fatality rate? To remind ourselves, here is the likelihood that you will 'survive the coronavirus' if you get it, in the view of Dr Simone Gold, of 'America's Frontline doctors':

Under age 20   survival rate 99.997%

Years 20 – 49   "   "   99.98%

Years 50 – 69   "   "   99.5%

Over 70 years   "   95%

- and those are the figures, without any treatment.[85] Thus if you're in the middle decades of twenty to fifty years of age, your chance of not recovering if you get CV19 'disease', is one in five thousand. (NB, Compare this with the graph given on page 26.)

No-one could be more qualified to have an opinion on this whole issue than Dr Michael Yeadon, the former Vice President of Pfitzer and its Chief Scientific advisor (also, founder and CEO of the biotech company Ziarco), and he affirmed in the summer of 2020:

> There is absolutely no need for vaccines to extinguish the pandemic... You do not vaccinate people who aren't at risk from a disease. You also don't set about planning to

---

[85] Simone Gold MD, 'The Truth about the covid-19 vaccine' (America's Frontline Doctors' 14.1.21 (on Bitchute) –risk vs age at 17 mins.

vaccinate millions of fit and healthy people with a vaccine that hasn't been extensively tested on human subjects.

The general public alas don't see it that way, having been effectively terrorised by government propaganda. As we've seen, the UK government spent over a hundred million pounds on a contract with one of the world's biggest advertising agencies made on March 2nd, 2020 i.e *several weeks before* the Lockdown was announced. The basic messages – to stay at home, wash your hands, etc – were thus agreed beforehand. Thereby we can appreciate the tremendous blitzkrieg of Lockdown propaganda we've all been experiencing.[86]

Strident Government propaganda aimed to overcome 'vaccine hesitancy.' That specific term was endorsed by the World Health Organization back in September 2019, as being a major threat to world health! The UK Government has mow contracted with a new advertising agency to work *for the next two years* in promoting its coronavirus story.[87] That company had already been promoting the usual message 'wash your hands, stay at home, keep your distance, wear a mask' – and will that continue for the next two years, until April 2023? That doesn't sound like the jab getting us back to normal. Do all 'pandemics' need expensive advertising campaigns?

What is happening now is at best a fascinating experiment, conducted on a population of volunteers, where nobody knows the outcome. Will it change Earth forever? Readers are advised to remain as observers rather than participants, as the effects may be irreversible.

Expected hazards relate primarily to death and infertility, with the latter only becoming evident after a year or two. To ascertain the former, the Office of National Statistics would merely have to publish its mortality data divided into those who have taken the

---

[86] Sott.net 'UK Govt struck 119 Covid advertising bill weeks before lockdown' *The Telegraph* 25.10.20
[87] 'Genesis appointed for Government Coronavirus Campaign' 20.3.21; on UK Government website as 'ID 3351409TEO-COVID: 'Hugo Talks' 18.3.21 'UK Govt book Covid advert Campaign until 2023!'

vaccine and those who have not. But, as they say, don't hold your breath.

The 'Vaccine' rollout started in December in the UK, followed a month later by hugely increased mortality figures. Dire stories started to emanate from nursing homes, from after they had been vaccinated. The graph shows over-80s mortality (data from NHS England), where, from the beginning of November to almost the end of January, we see a *trebling* of deaths (Its central line indicates 'first vaccine delivered' on December 8th)

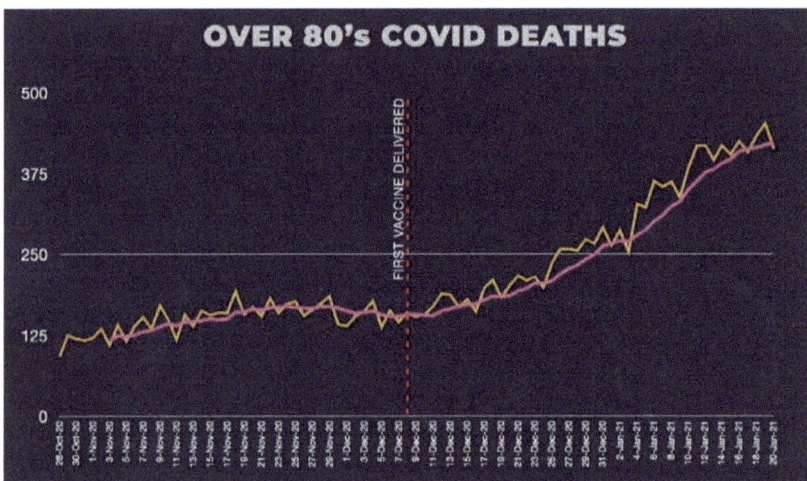

OVER 80's COVID DEATHS

Various talking heads soon appeared saying that correlation did not imply causality; which is indeed true, but if deaths shoot up once a vaccination program begins – and this is happening all over planet Earth – are we not entitled to some explanation? Cause and effect may be greatly muddled up here: When someone died within 60 or 28 days of a positive covid-19 test – however dubious the test result – they were automatically treated as a covid-19 death to push up the numbers. But when healthy young people die within hours of having a vaccination the deaths are dismissed as mere coincidences!

Dr Joseph Mercola commented upon this double standard:

Equally unjustifiable is the fact that death within months of a positive SARS-CoV-2 test was automatically pegged as a COVID-19 death, whereas death within days or even hours of the vaccine is shrugged off as coincidental, no matter how many times it happens. It is reprehensibly inexcusable the way these deaths are being attributed.'[88]

Deaths for 2020/1, England & Wales

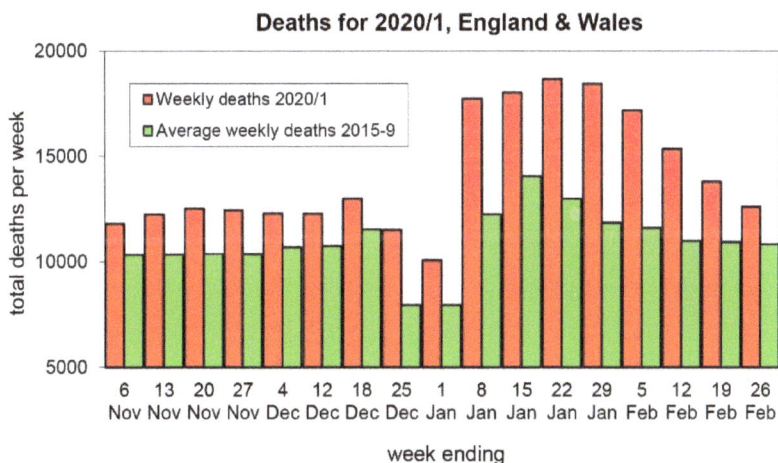

Here is a bar-chart showing weekly deaths in England & Wales for the start of 2021, comparing as before with the mean value for corresponding weeks from previous five years (ONS data). Suddenly, through January, 40% - 50% *more people were dying.* (NB a minimum in mortality over the Xmas period is here seen, which is quite normal and does not concern us). The week ending January 30th had eighteen thousand deaths as compared to twelve thousand average which is 55% more than expected, i.e. six thousand extra! What could have caused that?

Government experts started talking about a new 'strain' that had appeared, by way of accounting for this surge in mortality. In that case, people wondered, would the vaccine they had been given still work if a 'new strain' was abroad?

---

[88] Mercola,

Others wondered as to how, given that no lab had ever managed to isolate the Covid-19 virus, how could anyone tell that a new strain had appeared? Many were the gene-sequences of Covid-19 published in various countries, with the explanation given that it had kept 'mutating'. But how, if CV19 was mutating all of the time, could a 'new strain' have been detected? One noted an absence of attempts to demonstrate that a 'new strain' had appeared, or even to hint at how this might have been accomplished. There was talk about the alleged 'new strain' being '70% more infectious' which sounded rather bogus.

The surge in mortality following the vaccine was attributed to the 'virus'. Thus 'Bristol Live' reported on February 5th:

> Managers and staff at a Bristol care home have described how they did everything they could to keep coronavirus out – only for it to arrive just two weeks ago. Their valiant efforts kept the virus at bay for 11 months, until a sudden outbreak in the home in the third week of January – *after all the residents had been vaccinated.*

Ditto for an elderly care home in Germany where thirty-one healthy persons were vaccinated and eight died within weeks. The first died six days after being given it and the others about 14 days after. They had been given the 'BioNtech/Pfizer' vaccine. An eyewitness testified to *coercive* vaccinations: the vaccination team was accompanied by two soldiers, who they intimidated the elderly and undermined the will to resist. This was a retirement home in Berlin-Spandau.

Here is another such account from Spain:

> The Nuestra Señora del Rosario nursing home [in Andalusia] is reeling due to mass deaths after mRNA inoculations. All residents and workers at the facility received the first dose of Pfizer mRNA in early January, according to Spain mainstream media outlet ABC de Sevilla. Most residents became extremely ill shortly after

the shots. It is believed many came down with COVID-19, despite being vaccinated against it. The Andalusian Health Service reported that at least 46 residents have died since January. The situation remains dire . . .[89]

Many such reports are coming in, as alluded to in February 2021 by the group 'Doctors for COVID Ethics.' They sent an open letter to the European Medicines Agency (EMA) expressing concerns about what was happening:

> We note that a wide range of side effects is being reported following vaccination of previously healthy younger individuals with the gene-based COVID-19 vaccines. Moreover, there have been numerous media reports from around the world of care homes being struck by COVID-19 within days of vaccination of residents.

Historically, vaccine programs have a poor track record of reporting adverse reactions, with doctors not being mandated to report such. It is therefore encouraging to report an appeal by the 'UK Medical Freedom Alliance' -

> We believe that there is compelling evidence that the vaccines could be causing Covid-19 illness and deaths (Covid-19 and non-Covid-19 related) in certain cohoyrts. We therefore demand an urgent audit and full investigation of all the deaths that have occurred since the vaccine rollout began on 8 December 2020, to be carried out by scientists that are independent to SAGE and the Government and overseen by an All-Party Committee. We would like to see the results published publicly, before any rollout of second vaccine doses to those who have received the first dose.[90]

---

[89] Humansarefree.com 18.2.21 'Spain: Second Pfizer Shots Halted After 46 Nursing Home Residents Die After The First Shot'
[90] Open letter to Matt Hancock, November 2020, see ukmedfreedom.org

An article in the 'International Journal of Clinical Practice' in the autumn of 2020 reviewed previous coronavirus vaccine efforts[91] and found that for severe acute respiratory syndrome coronavirus (SARS-CoV), for Middle East respiratory syndrome coronavirus (MERS-CoV) and for respiratory syncytial virus (RSV), the vaccines had a tendency to trigger 'antibody-dependent enhancement'. Their disturbing conclusion was:

> COVID-19 vaccines designed to elicit neutralizing antibodies may sensitize vaccine recipients to more severe disease than if they were not vaccinated.

Experiments had earlier been done on ferrets because they apparently have very similar immune systems to humans. At first they seemed fine when given the mRNA, however months later on when such vaccinated animals were exposed to the virus a 'cytokine storm' developed and they mostly died. So, for CV19 they skipped the animal experiments. Will a whole new transhumanist entity start to appear, replacing the old humans? Legally vaccine manufacturers may be able to own humans who have synthetic nucleic acids in them.[92]

A top Belgian vaccines expert Geert Vanden Bossche, who has worked as an international vaccine developer, has warned[93] that, after millions have been vaccinated in just a few weeks, 'they will undoubtedly start to suffer from a steep incline in Covid-19 cases in the weeks to come. The steep decline we're seeing now may be followed by a short-lived plateau but a subsequent steep incline of (severe) diseases is inevitable.' This was he stressed an overall, population effect. That, in simple language, tends to support the prophetic words of Max Egon in February of 2021: 'Six months

[91] October 28, 'Disclosure to vaccine trial subjects of risk of COVID-19 vaccines Worsening Clinical disease', Cardozo & Veazey.
[92] Truthseeker.co.uk, Dr Carrie Madej 22.2.2012 'Future effects of those vaccinated,' 10 mins.
[93] Bitchute.com 'A Coming Covid Catastrophe' with Geert Vanden Bossche & Del Bigtree. 6.3.21.

down the track, we're going to see so many people getting ill from this vaccine.'

A group of twelve doctors sent a letter to the European Medical Association, expressing concern over serious potential consequences of COVID-19 vaccine technology. They warned of possible autoimmune reactions, blood clotting abnormalities, stroke and internal bleeding, "including in the brain, spinal cord and heart" and asked for assurances that each medical danger outlined "was excluded in pre-clinical animal models with all three vaccines prior to their approval for use in humans by the EMA." "Should all such evidence not be available", the authors wrote, "we demand that approval for use of the gene-based vaccines be withdrawn until all the above issues have been properly addressed by the exercise of due diligence by the EMA."[94]

Clearly, that won't happen, even though these new 'gene-based vaccines' have not been shown to be safe. Approval of the COVID-19 vaccines by the EMA was "premature and reckless", the doctors concluded: administration of the vaccines constituted and still does constitute "human experimentation", which was and still is "in violation of the Nuremberg Code,"

Formulated at the end of WW2, the *Nuremberg code* is a medical ethics guide which although not legally binding on anyone is widely respected. One of its principles states: 'No experiment should be conducted where there is an *a priori* reason to believe that death or disabling injury will occur.' Given what we know to-date, that principle is surely being violated right now by the 'vaccines' now being administered.

Are they Safe?

In place of any data on the long-term adverse effects of these new mRNA vaccines, we're just given a drumbeat of how year-by-year Covid vaccinations will become necessary:

---

94 Doctors4CovidEthics, 10th March.

Covid vaccines could become a regular part of winter – just like they are for flu, ministers have claimed. Revaccination against the illness is 'likely to become a regular part' of managing the disease, the Government has said. Scientists don't currently know how long vaccine-triggered immunity lasts for against Covid, given jabs were only created last spring. 'Over the longer term, revaccination is likely to become a regular part of managing Covid.[95]

Readers may here be reminded of Bill Gates' Microsoft Windows programs – surely the most virus-infested software ever - which kept needing new upgrades each year, whereby he acquired his fabulous wealth. The continuous upgrades sound very much like part of a transhumanist agenda: we'll refrain from further comment here, but in a year from now any new future that is appearing may start to become evident.

In March, 2021 the Council of Europe with 47 member-states[96] resolved that vaccines 'must not be mandatory' and that unvaccinated persons 'must not be discriminated against' - let's hope that edict is respected! In March 2021 Britain's Prime Minister seemed to be stating that vaccine passports would be required for international travel, with a majority of Britons apparently in agreement. It seems that 56% reckoned that such passports should be necessary for going to the pub or gym![97]

We just don't know the long-term side-effects of basically modifying people's DNA and RNA

stated Mark Zuckerburg, CEO of Facebook, in a video call to employees, in July of 2020. How true! Yet in December of 2020 Facebook adopted its official policy that it 'will remove any content

---

[95] Dailymail.co.uk 'revaccination may become a regular part of fighting the disease' March 2021.
[96] The UK remains a member, along with many non-EU states like Belarus, Russia and Turkey.
97 Yougov.co.uk 5 March 'Most Britons support a COVID-19 vaccine passport system.'

that claims Covid 19 vaccine changes people's DNA and RNA'! Subsequently his statement was leaked …

We're continually told how bad the 'covid-deniers' are, as their views are scrubbed so quickly from the Web. Here for example is ethical damnation from Bill Gates:

There are some things that are so extreme in terms of anti-vaccine or holocaust denial that you can draw a line, but how you draw that line and who is put in charge of that…[98]

Vaccine-sceptics are here equated with Holocaust deniers .. and Mr Gates wonders who will deal with them! Bearing in mind the $200 billion which Gates has made from his investment in vaccines over the last decade, such a view is understandable.[99]

As of March 4th the government had reported *a quarter of a million* injuries from taking the vaccine (based on its 'Yellow Card' scheme).

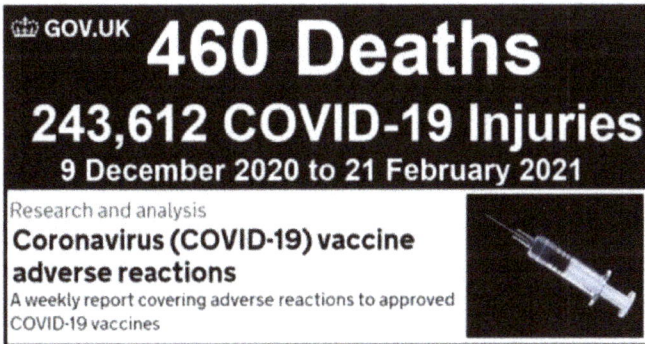

GOV.UK **460 Deaths**
243,612 COVID-19 Injuries
9 December 2020 to 21 February 2021
Research and analysis
Coronavirus (COVID-19) vaccine adverse reactions
A weekly report covering adverse reactions to approved COVID-19 vaccines

Israeli Experience

Israel has pursued a more intensive vaccination program than any other nation, with over half of its population getting the jab in a couple of months, using the Pfitzer vaccine. "Whoever does not get vaccinated will be left behind" its government is proclaiming. To

---

[98] www.rt.com/news/515902-bill-gates-three-vaccine-doses/ That quote is not findable on the web by any other means, than this *Russia Today* news page.
[99] Investing ten billion and receiving a 20:1 dividend: Bitchute, 'Bill Gates return on vaccines is $200 billion' 4.6.20, CNBC.

quote Gilad Atzmon, 'No-one can deny the astonishing fact that, in just 8 weeks of mass vaccination, the total number of Covid-19 deaths in the Jewish State almost doubled from the number accumulated in the prior ten months.' He added, 'The evidence collected in Israel points at a close correlation between mass vaccination, cases and deaths. This correlation points at the possibility that it is the vaccinated who actually spread the virus or even a range of mutants that are responsible for the radical shift in symptoms above.' We'll wait and see.

In Israel, An anti-vaxxer group known as "Anshei Emet" (People of Truth) has filed a suit against the Israeli government to the International Criminal Court (ICC), claiming is that 'many' have been killed, injured and severely damaged by the vaccine. The Health Ministry has "openly admitted that 41% of police persons, military, education and medical personnel who were vaccinated suffered severe side effects." This lawsuit is claiming that there are "no full reports of the numbers of dead or injured," despite data from clinical trials being released.

Their lawsuit argued that companies and associations that threatened to prevent unvaccinated employees from arriving to work were acting against the Nuremberg Code and that policies preventing unvaccinated people from receiving certain services and entering certain locations were against the code as well.

That sounds like a lawsuit worth following – although as Israel is

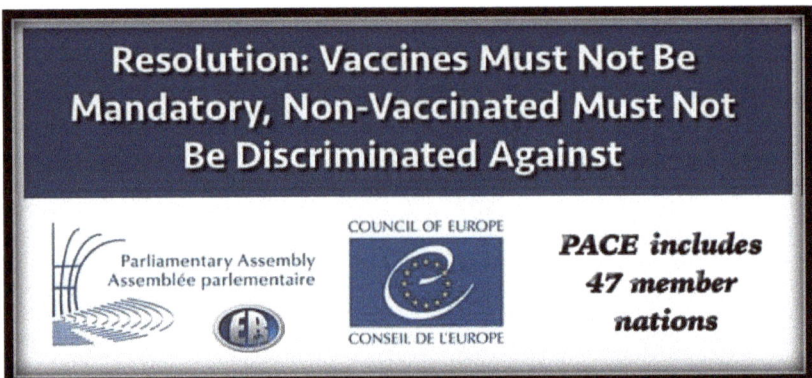

Resolution: Vaccines Must Not Be Mandatory, Non-Vaccinated Must Not Be Discriminated Against

Parliamentary Assembly
Assemblée parlementaire

COUNCIL OF EUROPE
CONSEIL DE L'EUROPE

PACE includes 47 member nations

not a signatory to the ICC it may not get very far. We are indeed not being given full reports of how many have died or been injured after taking the jab. Many are the newspaper reports which tell of people dying in old people's homes after being vaccinated and these need to be compiled together to obtain total figures.

Tanzania: the Heavy Price

Famously, President Magufuli of Tanzania sent for PCR-testing samples from a goat, motor oil, a papaya, a quail and a jackfruit. Four came back positive and one "inconclusive," which caused mirth all round the world. He banned the testing kits and called for an investigation into their origin and manufacture, dismissed a need for the new vaccines, dismissed CV19 as a Western hoax and started implementing naturopathic remedies for anyone suffering from Covid symptoms. His country Tanzania had only a very low incidence of 'covid' cases. His government was dedicated to health improvements and in consequence the life-expectancy of Tanzanians went up in each year of his presidency. Clearly, something had to be done.

The Guardian explained the need for action, with an article entitled, 'Its Time to Rein in Africa's anti-Vaxxer President' (5th Feb.), explaining how his policy was 'fuelling conspiracies and endangering lives' and therefore 'something had to be done.' 'He needs to be challenged openly and directly,' affirmed this anonymous author. The quite fit President Magufuli vanished two weeks later, soon after which he was announced dead of heart failure. He is reckoned to be the second African leader who died rather suddenly of heart failure, following their non-acceptance of the Covid narrative. That section of the *Guardian*, its 'Global Development' section, is sponsored by the Bill and Melinda Gates Foundation.[100] God bless you, Mr President.

---

[100] *Off-Guardian*, K.K., 'Tanzania –the Second Covid Coup?' 12.3.21

Conclusion

How could a minor disease killing an infinitesimal part of population (0.000045) have caused the collapse of civilization as we knew it?

Israel Shamir[101]

The inhabitants of Planet Earth agreed to take part in an experiment, by staying 'at home.' No-one had evidence that a lockdown procedure would help cure or remedy any new disease, if indeed it existed. But people agreed because of the potency of an image, that of a dire new virus that could somehow travel all around the world, and multiply and breed if it got inside you. After a couple of months, Mother Nature had enjoyed a marvellous unpolluted springtime and national economies had imploded, while in the USA overall mortality was remaining somewhat *lower* than in previous years –even though it had the world's highest number of C19 deaths?

The results of the great experiment are now in and enable the mortality figures to be compared with lockdowns. As we've already seen in previous chapters, the differing degrees of lockdown of various nations correlate *positively* with the degree of affliction by the alleged illness, measured as C19 deaths per million.

That is a common-sense result, because everyone knows that going out into the sunshine in the springtime is the best way to get rid of viral infections. And so it proved to be. The world's largest-scale experiment showed a general trendline: the less lockdown, the less C19 deaths.[102]

---

[101] Unz.com 'Coronavirus conspiracies' 22 May
[102] See Ch. 2, Iain Davies in the *Off-Guardian* commenting on 'The Oxford Coronavirus Government response Tracker.'

The result of this worldwide experiment has strikingly confirmed the message of a classic 2006 paper, 'Disease Mitigation Measures in the Control of Pandemic Influenza.'[103] British health experts need to read it. The legendary US doctor Donald Henderson, regarded as 'the twentieth century's most acclaimed disease eradicator'[104] was the moving force behind this paper. It argued *against* lockdown in the treatment of epidemics:

> There are no historical observations or scientific studies that support the confinement by quarantine of groups of possibly infected people for extended periods in order to slow the spread of influenza. ... It is difficult to identify circumstances in the past half-century when large-scale quarantine has been effectively used in the control of any disease. The negative consequences of large-scale quarantine are so extreme (forced confinement of sick people with the well; complete restriction of movement of large populations; difficulty in getting critical supplies, medicines, and food to people inside the quarantine zone) that this mitigation measure should be eliminated from serious consideration...

> Thus, cancelling or postponing large meetings would not be likely to have any significant effect on the development of the epidemic. While local concerns may result in the closure of particular events for logical reasons, a policy directing communitywide closure of public events seems inadvisable.

> Quarantine. As experience shows, there is no basis for recommending quarantine either of groups or individuals. The problems in implementing such measures are formidable, and secondary effects of absenteeism and community disruption as well as possible adverse consequences, such as loss of public trust in government and stigmatization of quarantined people and groups, are likely to be considerable....

and it concluded:

---

[103] *Biosecurity and Bioterrorism*, Vol 4, No. 4, 2006 by D.A. Henderson *et. al.*

Experience has shown that communities faced with epidemics or other adverse events respond best and with the least anxiety when the normal social functioning of the community is least disrupted. Strong political and public health leadership to provide reassurance and to ensure that needed medical care services are provided are critical elements. If either is seen to be less than optimal, a manageable epidemic could move toward catastrophe.

Ah, if only notice been taken of this paper! But people have nowadays grown so used to a diet of fear and being told what is the new enemy. They have actually become grateful for being told what to fear. It is a monster hoax which plays upon the fear of death itself, as this NHS poster shows:

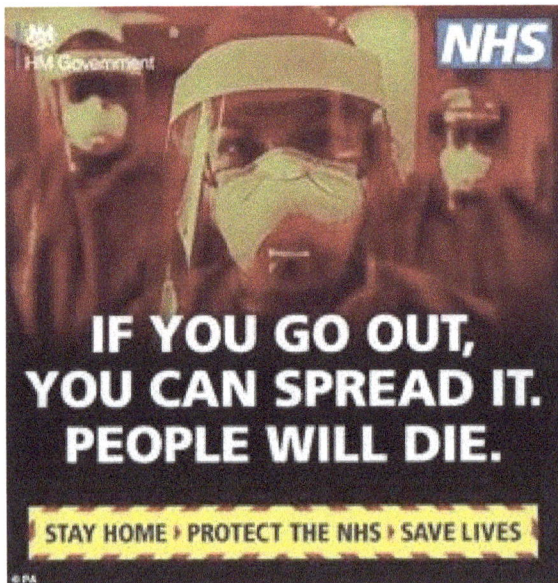

Figure: The Monster Hoax, NHS propaganda.

The contrary is the case. It is important to reject this suicide-

[104] American institute for economic Research, 'How a Free Society Deals with Pandemics, According to Legendary Epidemiologist and Smallpox Eradicator Donald Henderson' 21 May aeir.org; also jamesfetzer.org, Jeffrey A. Tucker, 'The 2006 Origins of the Lockdown Idea'

promoting, culture-extinguishing and nihilistic message.

Thus, a post-lockdown study by the financial giant JP Morgan shows *falling* infection rates since lockdowns were lifted in USA. Lockdowns have 'destroyed millions of livelihoods' its two authors concluded but they did not alter the course of the pandemic. The authors collated the virus R_0 rates (the rate at which infections are passed between people) in each US state and they compared the rates in each case on the day lockdown ended with the most recent R_0 measurement. They found that 'the vast majority of counties had decreased infection rates' after lockdowns were lifted.' The co-author of this study Marko Kolanovic - a trained physicist and a strategist for JP Morgan - said governments had been spooked by 'flawed scientific papers' into imposing lockdowns which were 'inefficient or late' and had little effect: 'Unlike rigorous testing of new drugs, lockdowns were administered with little consideration that they might not only cause economic devastation but potentially more deaths than Covid-19 itself.' Falling infection rates since lockdowns were lifted suggest they concluded that the virus 'likely has its own dynamics' which are 'unrelated to often inconsistent lockdown measures.' Many states showed a lower rate of transmission ('R') once the lockdown was ended.[105]

Again, this is just common sense, it's what one would expect.

A lot of people had believed in the lockdown, and that was because of their shared belief that a flu virus can be caught and transmitted. That is believed to happen by proximity, e.g from someone's breath if they coughed. People have been brought up to regard that as a common-sense view, and it attributes a terrific potency to any virus that is imagined to be present. People thereby imagine that their health can be undermined and death threatened by something invisible, over which they have no control. We've tried to argue here that they are *fearing the wrong thing:* rather one should

---

[105] Marko Kolanovic and Bram Kaplan 21 May; media reports of this survey on May 23rd did not allude to original paper.

fear the new 5G transmitters springing up everywhere plus one should also fear the new vaccine that threatens to turn us all into genetically modified organisms. No-one should fear a virus.

It was the Lockdowns that Killed people

We saw in Chapter One how a shocking peak in total UK mortality began *after* the lockdown. That turns out to be so, for *all* countries which imposed lockdowns and for which reliable death-data exists. Thus, we may be familiar with graphs such as this one as published by *The Economist,* showing a lockdown right after the increase began:

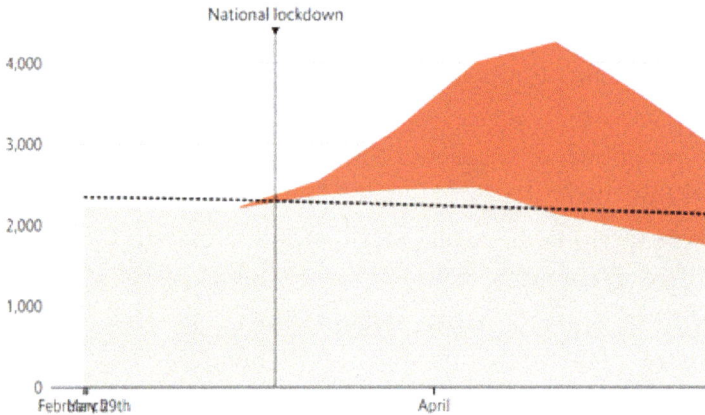

Belgium, confirmed weekly deaths

■ Deaths attributed to covid-19 ▦ All other deaths ······ Expected deaths

However, an insightful analysis on medium.com[106] demonstrated that it was the *first step* of Lockdown that was crucial. Thus while the above graph shows a March 18th date for 'the' national lockdown, there had been a phase one on March 13th that included widespread business closures. That was more exactly when the increase in mortality began, as the second graph shows. He checked six European nations plus the USA and Ecuador, and found that it was in each case the first-beginning date of Lockdown which started then mortality rise. Thus for the UK, on March 13th nursing homes started to ban visitors then on March 18 the closure of schools was

[106] 'Questions for Lockdown apologists' J. Pospichal, 23.5.20.

140

announced and on March 20 pubs, cafes and restaurants were closed. Finally the Government announced the full lockdown on the evening of March 23. In the UK we

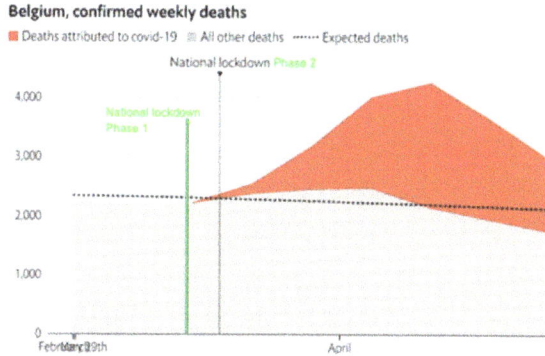

Belgium, confirmed weekly deaths
Deaths attributed to covid-19   All other deaths   ······ Expected deaths
National lockdown Phase 2

saw how the most reliable mortality data is weekly, from the Office of National Statistics. We saw in Chapter 1 how the increasing mortality in the UK just began to appear in the week prior to full lockdown (see graph on page 12), and now at last we can understand that. The conclusion to this study (by Mr Pospichal) is *so* important:

> We now have mortality data for the first few months of 2020 for many countries, and, as you might expect, there were steep increases associated with the beginning of the COVID-19 pandemic in each one. Surprisingly, however, these increases did not begin before the lockdowns were imposed, but after. Moreover, in almost every case, they began *immediately after*. Often, mortality numbers were on a *downward* trend before *suddenly reversing* course after lockdowns were decreed. Only after each country (or city) was locked down did the increases begin. Moreover, they began immediately, and in nearly every case, precipitously.
>
> All this leads us to the following questions, which we pose to all those who continue to defend the use of lockdowns as an effective means to prevent excess deaths.
>
> • Why was there *no* significant increase in overall mortality, in any country we have good data for, before the start of lockdowns?

- Why does a precise and exact correlation exist between the start of lockdowns and significant rises in overall mortality?

This is starting to look suspiciously like a mass murder program, a way of disposing of the elderly, sick and infirm, or a eugenics program to relieve government pension payouts.

We are in conclusion led to agree with the German legal council which has sought to bring 'the biggest class-action lawsuit in history', arguing that fraudulent PCR testing has been misused to engineer the appearance of a dangerous pandemic.[107] The lawsuit is based on the claim that '*SARS-CoV-2 'has not caused any excess mortality anywhere in the world,*' whereas pandemic measures have '*caused the loss of innumerable human lives, and have destroyed the economic existence of countless companies and individuals worldwide.*'[108] Both of those affirmations are correct.

Scientific method

A lot of what has gone catastrophically wrong in this story concerns the failure of normal and traditional scientific procedure. Our civilization has believed for centuries that practical and useful truth can be found using it. The scientific method can work provided that the livelihood of the investigator is not a factor in determining the required outcome. Nowadays massive corporate R&D has greatly overtaken that earlier process. Technology is developing, alarmingly, but does anyone still believe it is improving our lives? Those who advocate compulsory vaccination – where the doctor giving the jab literally doesn't know what it contains – claim to be pro-science. But science means *scientia*, knowledge. That knowledge might tell you that the virus does not as such exist, or not in the form in which it is imagined. It might tell us that giving the vaccine to a

[107] Seek for 'Reiner Fuellmich Crimes against Humanity.'
[108] A summary of this lawsuit was given by Dr Joseph Mercola in the journal *Nexus*, March 2021: 'The Covid-19 pandemic, The Greatest Hoax ever perpetrated on an unsuspecting public.'

142

few thousand consenting adults would be OK *as an experiment* - to ascertain whether, after the vaccination, they appeared more healthy or disease-resistant than the rest of the population? I think we all understand what the result would here be, and why that cannot be allowed to happen. Let's hear the words of professor Kurt Wittkowski about how traditional, scientific enquiry has been extinguished (more of this interview with *Spiked* online is quoted with kind permission in the Appendix):

> **Spiked:** Governments say they are following the science. Is that really true?
>
> **Wittkowski:** They have the scientists on their side that depend on government funding. One scientist in Germany just got $500million from the government, because he always says what the government wants to hear. Scientists are in a very strange situation. They now depend on government funding, which is a trend that has developed over the past 40 years. Before that, when you were a professor at a university, you had your salary and you had your freedom. Now, the university gives you a desk and access to the library. And then you have to ask for government money and write grant applications. If you are known to criticise the government, what does that do to your chance of getting funded? It creates a huge conflict of interest. The people who are speaking out in Germany and Switzerland are all independent of government money because they are retired.

A Survey

One-fifth of Britons believe the coronavirus story is a hoax! That's according to an Oxford University poll of two and a half thousand people at the beginning of May.[109] That is a good start. People are

---

[109] Freeman D., et al. (12 authors) *Psychological Medicine* 'Coronavirus conspiracy beliefs: mistrust and compliance with government guidelines' May 2020.

realising that some imposture has been put upon them. A much larger proportion, 59%, believe that *the government is misleading them* about the whole affair. We are indeed living in a world where people are no longer able to trust 'the glib and oily art' with which politicians speak. 62% agree 'to some extent that the virus is man-made' vis a vis the original form of the virus having been prepared in US Bio-labs - which probably is the case.

When asked whether they believed that coronavirus is a bio-weapon developed by China to destroy the West, 55 per cent said they did not agree, and again this shows the good sense of the British people, for that is surely not the case. Only 5% agreed with this nutty notion. Then 79% said they did not agree that coronavirus is caused by 5G. Again that is a correct judgment: 5G is a surely major contributing factor towards what is being experienced as the C19 pandemic, but it should not be viewed as 'the cause.'

So altogether the results of this survey of the British people are quite encouraging. Let's hope that in due course they come to accept the view of the *Washington Times'* editorial of 26th April:

> COVID-19 will go down as one of the political world's biggest, most shamefully overblown, overhyped, overly and irrationally inflated and outright deceptively flawed responses to a health matter in American history.

Or maybe as an even better one-sentence final judgment we should quote from the excellent article 'lockdown Lunacy the thinking person's guide' on childrenshealthdefence.org

> Knowing what we know today about COVID-19's Infection Fatality Rate, asymmetric impact by age and medical condition, non-transmissibility by asymptomatic people and in outdoor settings, near-zero fatality rate for children, and the basic understanding of viruses through Farr's law, locking down society was a bone-headed policy decision so devastating to society that historians may judge it as the all-

time worst decision ever made.

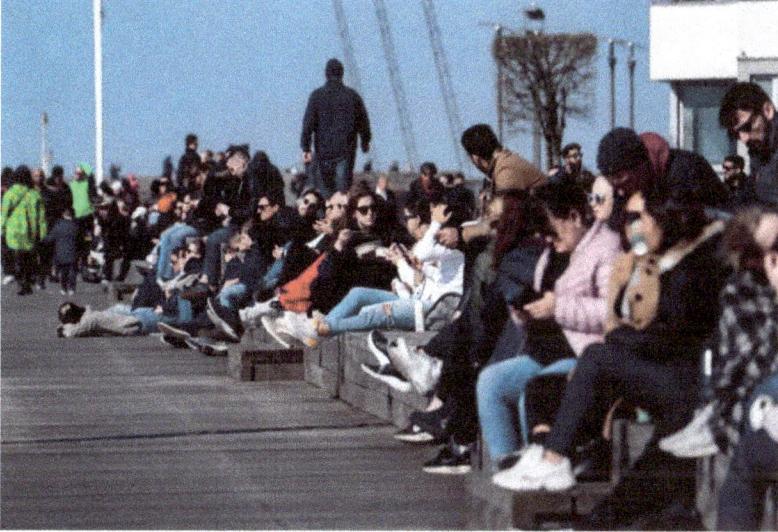

Figure: relaxed citizens of Malmo in Sweden, on April 14th

Sweden, it seems, was right. They are emerging from this crisis with confidence and optimism. Here to conclude is an image of people in Malmo on April 14th having a good time, when the rest of the West was in lockdown.

Daily New Deaths in Sweden

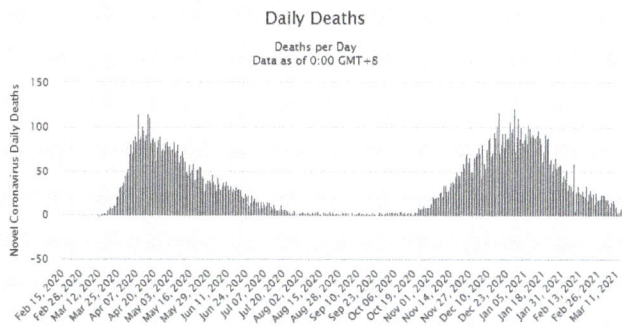

Figure: Coronavirus 'daily deaths' in Sweden: peaking in April then extinct by July, followed by a 'second wave' in December-January. worldometers.info

Appendix

1. Swiss Policy Research conclusions[110]

A good web-page for reference.

1. According to the latest immunological and serological studies, the overall lethality of Covid-19 (IFR) is about 0.1% and thus in the range of a strong seasonal influenza (flu).

2. In countries like the US, the UK, and also Sweden (without a lockdown), overall mortality since the beginning of the year is in the range of a strong influenza season; in countries like Germany, Austria and Switzerland, overall mortality is in the range of a mild influenza season.

3. Even in global "hotspots", the risk of death for the general population of school and working age is typically in the range of a daily car ride to work. The risk was initially overestimated because many people with only mild or no symptoms were not taken into account.

4. Up to 80% of all test-positive persons remain symptom-free. Even among 70-79 year olds, about 60% remain symptom-free. Over 95% of all persons develop at most moderate symptoms.

5. Up to 60% of all persons may already have a certain cellular background immunity to Covid-19 due to contact with previous coronaviruses (i.e. common cold viruses). The initial assumption that there was no immunity against Covid-19 was not correct.

6. The median age of the deceased in most countries (including Italy) is over 80 years (e.g. 86 years in Sweden) and only about 4% of the deceased had no serious preconditions. The age and risk profile of deaths thus essentially corresponds to normal mortality.

7. In many countries, up to two thirds of all extra deaths occurred in nursing homes, which do not benefit from a general lockdown. Moreover, in many cases it is not clear whether these people really died from Covid19 or from weeks of extreme stress and isolation.

---

[110] swprs.org/a-swiss-doctor-on-covid-19/

8. Up to 30% of all additional deaths may have been caused not by Covid19, but by the effects of the lockdown, panic and fear. For example, the treatment of heart attacks and strokes decreased by up to 60% because many patients no longer dared to go to hospital.

9. Even in so-called "Covid19 deaths" it is often not clear whether they died *from* or *with* coronavirus (i.e. from underlying diseases) or if they were counted as "presumed cases" and not tested at all. However, official figures usually do not reflect this distinction.

10. Many media reports of young and healthy people dying from Covid19 turned out to be false: many of these young people either did not die from Covid19, they had already been seriously ill (e.g. from undiagnosed leukaemia), or they were in fact 109 instead of 9 years old. The claimed increase in Kawasaki disease in children also turned out to be false.

2. Voices of Dissent

A. Ontario doctor Mark Trozzi   March 2021

Trozzi. He had practiced has practiced Emergency Medicine for the past twenty-five years, but his conscience has obliged him to resign from his very lucrative job.

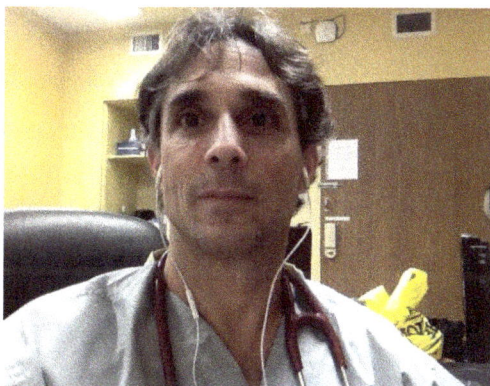

Figure: what an honest doctor looks like – Dr Mark Trozzi.

"The "first wave" of the "pandemic" was absolutely the quietest time in my career. I have worked very hard and been very busy over the past twenty-five years in the ER ['Emergency Room']. However, both in my regular ER and my "COVID-19 designated" ER, there were almost no patients, and almost no work. I had multiple long ER shifts without a single patient.

"Meanwhile, when I would go to the local grocery store, the propagandized public, God bless them, would usher me to the front of the antisocial distance line, thanking me for everything I was going through as a front-line emergency doctor.

They believed that the ER's and hospitals were full of patients dying from covid, and that I must be exhausted and at risk of dying myself from exposure. I began contacting doctors and friends all over Canada and the US, and found the same pattern: empty hospitals, and propaganda saying that they were full of patients dying of covid.

Early in my studies, I investigated zinc and hydroxychloroquine, which based on sound physiology, may genuinely help those rare persons who get very sick with this cold virus. I was surprised that this treatment was simply brushed aside and dismissed by most of the medical community.

At every level, hospital administration has had no apparent choice, other than to submit to the endless top-down roll out from governments, of questionable new rules, protocols, and procedures.

I have never seen a patient sick with COVID-19; I have seen some positive PCR tests in asymptomatic people, and watched people be imprisoned in their own homes and isolated from family and friends.

My research into the PCR test has convinced me personally that it is misleading, manipulatable, and being used to drain endless taxpayer's money and future debt, to dramatically enrich the very criminals running this scandal.

"My province alone has performed ~50,000 PCR tests daily. Meanwhile our federal government is bringing in hundreds of thousands of doses of potentially dangerous experimental injections of modified viral genetic material, calling them "vaccines", and having the military manage them. Is this reasonable for a predominantly mild and non-fatal viral illness.

I have watched the suppression of doctors and scientists who performed serum antibody studies, whose findings showed that the virus was much more widespread, yet generally nonfatal, and asymptomatic or very mild in most cases; and that in many regions we had likely already achieved natural herd immunity by summer 2020.

"I perceive that many things we learned in medical school about infectious disease, have been brushed aside and replaced by constantly expanding lists of often ******* mandates by public health officials. Doctors, nurses, and teachers are especially important to the success of this COVID-19 deception, as we are leaders in society and people trust our advice.

"There are many positive and negative motivators being used to manipulate Canadian doctors, nurses and teachers, to inadvertently participate in this grand covid deception; but this is destroying our society. Much of what is being done, including the experimental viral genetic injections, seem to violate the Nuremberg code regarding medical experimentation with full informed consent by the participants. Doctor's and nurses face tough decisions. My career as an emergency physician always provided me an opportunity to practice my religious and ethical beliefs of honesty and kindness, while making a good living. Now maintaining the career I love, would require participating in the deception, violating my oath and spiritual beliefs, and in my opinion committing crimes against humanity as defined by the Nuremberg Code.

"The forced wearing of masks by most of the world's population is not unanimously supported by real science. These masks cause significant harm to our psychological, social, dermatological and dental health. Though I generally have great health, the masks have given me rashes and nasal symptoms whenever I have had to wear them for prolonged periods, which resolve whenever I do not wear them for a few days. What I find most disturbing is the elimination of facial expressions, and hence normal visual social interaction.

"The history of past attempts at vaccines for coronaviruses, revealed some very dangerous side effects in animal models, and the efforts were abandoned. Why would we take a dangerous vaccine for a generally mild illness, to which we develop herd immunity anyway? The current roll-out of fast-tracked expensive experimental "vaccines" is burying the taxpayers in endless debt to the rich and powerful villains of this story. Yet, we the people who have been imprisoned and abused in this scandal, are being manipulated into taking new strange injections, in hopes that we might regain some of our freedom. Additionally the so called "vaccines" are not vaccines (unless we change the definition of vaccines). Rather they are injections of Corona-virus genes. They are covid-19 genetic material, a modified part of the covid-19 virus's genetic code.

They are advertised to enter your cells, engage with and use your ribosomes which normally produce only your own cell's complex parts or "proteins" based on your genetic code and your messenger RNA. Naturally, inside your cells, your messenger-RNAs bring your many natural proteins' designs from their hard-copy within your DNA, to your cells' ribosomes outside of the nucleus. Hence your messenger-RNA normally carry elements of your genetic code from your DNA that is within your cells' nuclei, to your ribosomes, which read the codes and produce your cellular machinery called "proteins". However, when the ribosomes are engaged by the viral messenger RNA injection, your cells start producing part of the virus: the viral "spike glycoprotein of SARS-CoV-2". So this is where it starts to have some relationship to vaccines, but it's very different. Here, your own cells have viral genes inside, directing them to spend nutrients and energy to produce and pump out copies of part of the covid-19 virus into your circulation..."

We should agree with Henry Makow, "There is only one courageous honest doctor in Ontario, who takes the Hippocratic Oath seriously." Let's compare that with personal testimony from a UK hospital worker:

"I have been a porter in one of the largest hospitals in the UK for the past three years. I have never experienced the hospital so quiet as in the last 12 months. The MSM has painted a false narrative which has, in the main, been universally accepted by the public at large. The ICU has indeed been busy, with co-morbidity ('covid') patients and little else. I have seen both bays closed and whole wards shut down - because they were not needed. There is no requirement to "protect the NHS" as it is like a ghost town - understandably the general public do not want to be there. The real issue is that due to the illogical dictates by the british government, many staff have had to isolate (needlessly) - thus resulting in staff shortages. I saw a patient at one end of a corridor (with a nurse) talking to a relative at the other end, about 20 meters away - they hadn't seen each other for twelve months and were allowed no physical contact. This is one of many crimes against humanity that is being perpetrated on a daily basis. The only epidemic here is one of intentional fear, deception, coercion and manipulation by the players in this unfolding scenario. And yet this is only the beginning."

One has heard many stories of this nature.

B. Vernon Coleman, 'Coronavirus &Why you are now in great danger' 15th April 2020

Knowing that nowhere near enough people are dying of the CV to justify the oppressive measures they have introduced, the authorities are quietly making sure that most of the people who die are (or at least a large proportion) being classified as coronavirus deaths. Indeed there is some evidence that people are being classified as CV victims without ever having been tested. And it seems that Britain is doing what the Italians did: if a patient has the virus and they die, then they died of the virus. But I suspect Britain's going one step further: if someone who dies is thought to have had the virus, or might have had the virus, then they are CV victims and their death is added to the total. The lack of any testing or any real extensive testing makes this easy. Today it is clear to me and to a lot of other people that the cure not the problem is causing this crisis....

CV certainly appears as far less deadly than the flu. Fiddling the figures is the final cruel deceit to sustain the fear and to excuse the new totalitarian tactics being used to keep us all quiet. Meanwhile its now acknowledged that the number of people who died as a direct result of the restrictions brought in by governments will far exceed the number of people who will die as a result of the CV. The British government has now admitted that the side-effects of the cure, the lockdown and so on, will result in 150,000 unnecessary deaths in the UK. No-one is now suggesting that there will be anything like that number of deaths from the CV...

Scientists are now wedded to this deceit. Even if they wanted to, how could they possibly ever admit that they got it so very, very wrong? ..

No-one seems now to have any idea of how they are going to get out of the lockdowns, how are they going to stop them, how are they going to get rid of the fear? How are they going to stop people from being terrified of a virus, which is still going to exist, when the lockdown has ended? The evidence that the CV has been exaggerated is all around us.

The NHS has 2,295 empty intensive care-beds. The average number of empty intensive care beds before the CDV crisis was 800. So the NHs has 1,495 more empty intensive-care beds during the CV crisis than it did before the so-called crisis began. Obviously these figures keep changing. It's been reported that almost half of the beds in some English hospitals are lying empty. We're heading for a manufactured CV apocalypse.

Vernon Coleman, as an elderly, widely-published and respected voice on health and nutrition, was startled to find that his popular videos on the topic had all been deleted. In an interview reflecting upon this, he states: 'I don't think anyone in government now denies that the number of people dying because of the lockdowns, the so-called 'cure' for the coronavirus, will be far, far greater than the number who will die from the virus itself... Everything I've written recorded about the coronavirus has resulted in my reputation being trashed, so much that I'd have been far better off if I'd kept my thoughts to myself.'[111] We're glad he didn't!

****

c. An anonymous expert on microbiology.

"What the Chinese have done is sequence a nucleic acid in some material they suspected but did not confirm of causing antibiotic-resistant pneumonia, And pneumonia due to air pollution is well known to be an actual epidemic in China, especially Wuhan, which saw vigorous air pollution protests in the summer of 2019.

Of course, the PCR tests used in China (and everywhere else, for many purposes) are widely known to be neither precise nor reliable. Patients test positively if the genetic sequence of their blood or

---

[111] Vernon Coleman, 'Why did Youtube ban my video?' 13 May.

respiratory tract sample has a "high degree" of similarity with that of the virus. Reports of 80% false positives in "asymptomatic individuals" and recovered patients were reported from China at that time

The creator of the PCR test, Kary Mullis, who died perhaps not uncoincidentally on 12th August 2019, long ago acknowledged it could not work for the purposes for which it is routinely used in medical science. [That death is certainly tragic, because everyone would have wanted to hear the view of that lucid and honest Nobel-prize winning biochemist on this topic. Concerning the date of his death, it was one day before the big *Operation Crimson Contagion* began - NK]

In the US, the Centers for Disease Control (CDC) issued guidance to health care professionals, widely reported, as of March 24: "COVID-19 should be reported on the death certificate for all decedents where the disease caused or is assumed to have caused or contributed to death." The new diagnostic code was in actuality issued to the CDC by the World Health Organization (WHO) "for clinical or epidemiological diagnosis of COVID-19 where a laboratory confirmation is inconclusive or not available…"

New York City hospitalization and death figures of 29,335 and 6,182 respectively as of April 13 continue to defy the on-the-ground reality seen at empty local hospitals and unverified reports of overflowing morgues … ultimately, tracking people appears to be the goal, despite the fact that no virus has been identified, isolated, or proven to cause a disease known as COVID-19.

In the UK, elderly individuals and the parents of sick children have been asked to sign "do not resuscitate" orders so as to make room for alleged COVID patients.' ('When a Pandemic becomes a Shamdemic' by 'regensordo,' therulingclassobserver.com + Jim Fetzer's blog 14th April)

****

D. 'Perspectives on the Pandemic' by prof Knut Wittkowski. This popular and informative video was deleted by Youtube. For 20 years Wittkowski was head of the Biostatistics, Epidemiology and Research

Design department at the Rockefeller University's Centre for Clinical Science, and earlier he had been at Tubingen University. He is exactly the sort of expert the government should have consulted, if it had wished for a humane and caring response. Instead he had his Youtube videos deleted. Social distancing and lockdown he here argues are the worst way to deal with an airborne respiratory virus:

'When flu strikes, there is a need to protect the elderly: whereas children do very well with these diseases, they are evolutionarily designed to be exposed to all sorts of viruses, during their lifetime, and so they should keep going to schools and infecting each other, which contributes to herd immunity, which means that after about four weeks at the most, the elderly can start rejoining the family because the virus will have been extinguished.

Will containment prolong the duration of the virus?   "With all respiratory diseases, the only thing that stops the disease is herd immunity. About 80% of the people need to have had contact with the virus, and the majority of them won't even recognise that they had been infected, or they just get very, very mild symptoms, especially if they are children. So its very important to keep the schools open, and kids mingling, and spread the virus, to get herd immunity as fast as possible, and then the elderly people, who should be separated can come back when the virus has been exterminated.

Is it a policy to contain everybody? "Its not the first coronavirus that comes out and it won't be the last. For all respiratory diseases we have the same type of epidemic: if you leave it alone, it comes for two weeks, it peaks, and it goes for two weeks, then its gone."
Staying indoors "Keeps the virus healthy. Going outdoors stops every respiratory illness."
Prof Wittkowski has come out with the only memorable line in this whole affair: 'We could open up again and forget the whole thing.' Here is a part of the *Spiked* interview (quoted with kind permission) in which

he said this.

spiked Is Covid-19 dangerous?

Knut Wittkowski: No, unless you have age-related severe comorbidities. So if you are in a nursing home because you cannot live by yourself anymore, then getting infected is dangerous.

spiked: How far along is the epidemic?

Wittkowski: It is over in China. It is over in South Korea. It is substantially down in most of Europe and down a bit everywhere, even in the UK. The UK and Belarus are latecomers, so you do not see exactly what you are seeing in continental Europe. But everywhere in Europe, the number of cases is substantially declining.

spiked: Have our interventions made much of an impact?

Wittkowski: When the whole thing started, there was one reason given for the lockdown and that was to prevent hospitals from becoming overloaded. There is no indication that hospitals could ever have become overloaded, irrespective of what we did. So we could open up again, and forget the whole thing. I hope the intervention did not have too much of an impact because it most likely made the situation worse.

The ideal approach would be to simply shut the door of the nursing homes and keep the personnel and the elderly locked in for a certain amount of time, and pay the staff overtime to stay there for 24 hours per day.

spiked: Are we on the way to reaching herd immunity?

Wittkowski: All the studies that have been done have shown that we already have at least 25 per cent of the population who are immune. That gives us a nice cushion. If 25 per cent of the population are already immune, we are very quickly getting to the 50 per cent that we need to have what is called herd immunity.

spiked: Should we worry about a second spike?

Wittkowski: This is an invention to justify a policy that politicians are afraid of reversing.

spiked: Should people practice social distancing?

Wittkowski: No.

spiked: Why not?

Wittkowski: Why? What is the justification for that? People need to ask the government for an explanation. The government is restricting freedom. You do not have to ask me for justification.

spiked: How did we get this so wrong?

Wittkowski: Governments did not have an open discussion, including economists, biologists and epidemiologists, to hear different voices. In Britain, it was the voice of one person – Neil Ferguson – who has a history of coming up with projections that are a bit odd. The government did not convene a meeting with people who have different ideas, different projections, to discuss his projection. If it had done that, it could have seen where the fundamental flaw was in the so-called models used by Neil Ferguson.. The assumption was that one per cent of all people who became infected would die. There is no justification anywhere for that.

Knowing that the epidemic would be over in three weeks, and the number of people dying would be minor, just like a normal flu, the governments started shutting down in mid-March. Why? Because somebody pulled it out of his head that one per cent of all infected would die. One could argue that maybe one per cent of all *cases* would die. But one per cent of all people infected does not make any sense. And we had that evidence by mid-March.

spiked: Just to clarify, cases are different from people infected?

Wittkowski: Cases means people who have symptoms that are serious enough for them to go to a hospital or get treated. Most people have no symptoms at all. But waking up with a sore throat one day is not a case. A case means that someone showed up in a hospital.

E. Others:

* Professor **Sucharit Bhakdi** a medical microbiologist and infectious disease epidemiologist asked: 'To gauge the true danger of the virus, what is the type of information we need?' and his answer was, to compare the effect of CV-19 with the common corona viruses 'that we live with every day.' A comparison had been made of ten thousand patients 'all with respiratory track diseases that are infected with common corona viruses; and then another ten thousand such cases infected with CV-19'. The mortality was no different between the two groups. He was alluding to a French study published 19th March[112] (theblogmire.com/ 22nd March)

* **Dr John Lee** The Spectator 28 March 'How Deadly is the Coronavirus?': "We have yet to see any statistical evidence for excess deaths, in any part of the world... the vast majority of respiratory deaths in the UK are recorded as bronchopneumonia, pneumonia, old age or a similar designation... Of the people dying in the first three months of this year, globally, the CV cases represent 0.14%; These figures might shoot up but they are, right now, lower than other infectious diseases that we live with (such as flu)"

* **Prof John Oxford** is a leading UK virology expert who runs a secure isolation ward for testing treatments for viruses. On 31st March 2020 he denounced what he said was a 'media epidemic' where COVID-19 was less harmful than a normal flu season. He describes it as 'the greatest exercise in Groupthink folly this country has ever witnessed.'

****

3. 5G and the Elusive Safety Threshold

We'd all like to be reassured that there is some kind of 'safety threshold' for the new microwave radiation. The government has indeed got one, but is it a million times too high? To keep things simple we use only these two units: $\mu W /Cm^2$ or $\mu W /m^2$. The latter, microwatts per square metre, is ten thousand times smaller or weaker than the

---

[112] 'SARS-CoV-2: fear versus data', Int Jnl of Antimicrobial Agents Roussel et. Al., 19 March

former, microwatts per square centimetre.

Public Health England accept the safety threshold of twenty watts per square meter. That is used for example by Ofcom, in assuring us that school playgrounds are perfectly safe. We can write this as 20,000,000 $\mu W/m^2$ or as 2,000 μW /cm^2. (A microwatt is a millionth of a watt). Ofcom was happy to report that school playgrounds scored a mere 1% of the official safe limit, so it was OK. They would have used a metre like the one shown here, for this purpose. So the UK school playground levels are found to average around 200,000 $\mu W/m^2$ of electromagnetic radiant energy.

The instructions for that 'Acoustimeter' state[113]: 'The German Building Biology Institute recommend no higher than 10 $\mu W/m^2$ for only slight effects (though for electrosensitive people even less than this creates a problem), with 'severe' set at 1000 $\mu W/m^2$. It gives a safety threshold 'only slight effects' of 70 $\mu W/m^2$. Those safe levels are several orders of magnitude lower than what has been found in school playgrounds.

Here is the view of British expert Oliver Perceval: "Many International long-term biological guidelines recommend only 0.1-100 $\mu W/m^2$ (microwatts per square metre) as the long-term exposure limit

---

113 It refers to https://stop5g.co.uk/safe-levels-non-ionising-radiation/

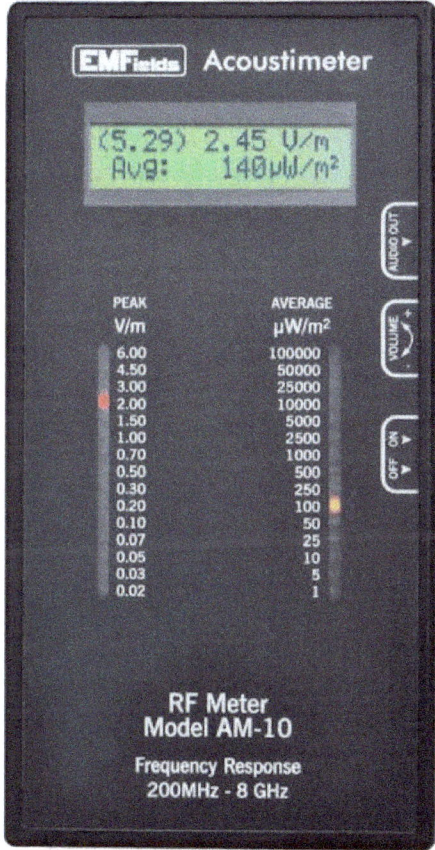

for biological effect prevention….In many public areas and streets in the UK the levels are now around 250 μW/m² on a constant basis." He has described the government guidelines[114] as 'completely inadequate and inappropriate' for protecting the populace.

Here is the view of Barry Trower concerning modern schools: 'I have always predicted that any school which allows itself to be 'bathed' in microwaves from whatever source will see its sicknesses rise and behaviour fall. I have received many phone calls to confirm this. In all of the schools I have visited around the world with WI-FI, every one has reported the same symptoms in students: fatigue, headaches, nausea,

---

114 These derive from the International Commission on Non-Ionizing Radiation Protection (ICNIRP).

chest pain, vision problems.'[115]

We turn to the 'Bio-Initiative 2012, A Rationale for Biologically-based Exposure standards for low-intensity EM Radiation' (https://bioinitiative.org/conclusions/) It found:

* Various cell tower studies report bioeffects in the range of 3 to 500 $\mu W/m^2$

* Human sperm damaged by cell phone radiation between 3.4 to 700 $\mu W/m^2$.

* Child & adolescent headaches, sleep disturbance and concentration difficulties 10-100 $\mu W/m^2$

It concluded that "Public safety standards are 1,000 – 10,000 or more times higher than levels now commonly reported in mobile phone base station studies to cause bioeffects" and it suggested a threshold value of 3 $\mu W/m^2$ as a reasonable for protecting a population.[116] Based on this the UK government's safety threshold is *a million times* too high.

Chapter 6 has recommended the Firstenberg masterpiece *The Invisible Rainbow,* but that did not however discuss safety levels. It may be studied in conjunction with the excellent site, 'bioinitiative.org.'

A guide for home building entitled 'Create Healthy Homes' is useful for couples wanting to have children. Here is its view: 'The building biology profession and EMF experts around the world say 10 microWatts per meter squared or less is safe for sleeping areas (actually, 0.1 $\mu W/m^2$ is our "No Anomaly" level for sleeping areas).'[117]

It's the usual story: HM Government is in bed with Big Business and endorses its 'safety thresholds.' These may be OK for industrial workers as long as they don't want to breed but are criminally negligent as regards child exposure to EM radiation. The Government says 'I can trust you, can't I?' and Big Business says 'Yes of course you can.' The government then becomes unable to back down on reassurances it has given, for fear of ensuing lawsuits. What this country needs is an Environmental Protection Agency that does *not* have a revolving door

---

[115] From Trower's 'Declaration' given to a US District court in 2011
116 For these threshold values outlined, see video '5G Apocalypse as the Extinction event' at 20 mins.
[117] https://createhealthyhomes.com/bb_standards.php

with Big Pharma or electronic industries nor is funded by them, that *is* based on real biological science experimentation, and *can* modify and adjust its recommended safety thresholds as new evidence comes along, on a no-guilt, no-blame basis.

Biblio

Corona, False alarm? Facts and Figures 2020 Reiss and Bhakdi   (an Amazon bestseller)

Fear of the Invisible, 2008, Janine Roberts

Goodbye Germ Theory: ending a Century of Medical Fraud 2008 Dr W Trebing

The Contagion Myth, why Viruses (including "Coronavirus") are not the cause of disease 2020 Cowan & Morell (banned by Amazon)

The Invisible Rainbow A History of Electricity and Life 2016 Arthur Firstenberg

Virus Mania, How the Medical industry continually invents Epidemics 2007 Engelbrecht & Kohnlein

Index

www.ingramcontent.com/pod-product-compliance
Lightning Source LLC
Chambersburg PA
CBHW041220030426
42336CB00024B/3402